Distributed in the United States of America and Canada
by Howell Book House Inc.
230 Park Avenue, New York, N.Y. 10169

Published in Great Britain by
Collins Professional Books
8 Grafton Street, London W1X 3LA
First published 1987
Copyright © Mary Bromiley 1987

Printed and bound in Great Britain by
Mackays of Chatham, Kent

British Library Cataloguing in Publication Data
Bromiley, Mary W.
  Equine injury and therapy
  Horses–Wounds and injuries
  I. Title
  636.1′08971   SF951

ISBN 0–87605–864–0

Equine Injury and Therapy

Mary W. Bromiley
MCSP, SRP, RPT (USA)
Chartered Physiotherapist

Drawings by Penelope Slattery
Photography by Jennifer Slattery
and Tom McQuilton

HOWELL BOOK HOUSE INC.
230 Park Avenue, New York, N.Y. 10169

Foreword

Of all the equestrian sports the three day event is probably the most exacting, resulting at times in a variety of different injuries to the horse. Sometimes these injuries can be superficial, with the horse 'back on the road' within twenty-four hours. Sometimes they can be more serious with the horse being laid off for a year or longer. Looking back over more than twenty years of competitive riding, my horses seem to have suffered injuries mostly resulting in the horses, and my sporting aspirations, being confined to their stable or field for months on end.

Nowadays, with human medicine increasingly being adapted and applied to veterinary medicine, we are able to rapidly accelerate the natural healing process. This means injuries that used to take months to heal can now be remedied in weeks. Not only can the healing be speeded up but now many chronic conditions can be avoided if they are caught in time.

Mary Bromiley has been in the forefront of these advances for many years. The daughter of a man who was both vet and doctor, a highly successful 'West End' physiotherapist, few people can have been better qualified. She has used her skills and machines in human medicine to develop a highly successful horse practice. The road to success has not been easy, often blocked by the traditionalists advocating extended rest or old fashioned remedies. She is a highly practical, no-nonsense person, motivated by her own experience and convictions.

My horses and I have been lucky enough to know Mary Bromiley for three years, and to reap the benefit of her expertise. I would recommend to anyone her refreshingly modern and practical approach to the healing of horse injuries.

Whatever your interests with horses, as owner or rider, in racing or competition, in hunting or hacking, this book will help you to understand your horse and what you can do to help him if he is injured. In some cases you can help improve performance and help prevent injury.

Whether you see the horse as athlete, friend, or both, this book makes very worthwhile reading.

Captain Mark Phillips

Acknowledgements

My grateful thanks go to the members of the veterinary profession who have trusted me with their patients, and to all the owners, trainers and head lads who, over the years, have given me support and help by allowing me to work with them and their horses.

My thanks also to my secretary Manou Koch de Gooreynd, who has deciphered my writing and typed the original manuscript.

1 The Musculoskeletal System Explained

The concept of treatment and rehabilitation following athletic injury is an acceptable part of human medicine and is the task of the physiotherapist. The physiotherapist is part of a team, a team headed by the doctor in charge of the case. The doctor makes the initial diagnosis and writes a prescription requesting treatment for the condition ascribed to the patient.

Originally, the physiotherapist had only his/her hands and the ability of the patient to perform specific tasks under direction. With the arrival of the machine era, the physiotherapist learned of the effects, on tissue, of these machines. An in-depth knowledge of anatomy and physiology allowed for the choice of the machine most appropriate for the condition diagnosed, and furthermore the ability to change machines as the recovery pattern required.

Therapy machines have, in the main, been developed for use in the human field, with no adaptations for use in veterinary medicine other than reshaping pads and changing names – for example, an ultrasonic machine has been renamed a vetsonic. It must be understood that no clinical trials have been run or are running to ascertain the exact effects of these human-orientated machines on the tissues of the horse. However, fractures, sprains, strains, arthritis, muscle tears, bruising, painful backs, are all common to human and horse, and the machines are being widely used to treat athletic injuries of both horse and rider.

Unfortunately, little has been written for the layman describing the best way to use the machines, the dangers of overdosage or the contra-indications, the only available literature being the manufacturers' pamphlets or books written for members of the medical or veterinary profession, requiring an in-depth, specialist knowledge. In an ideal world, only the professionals should use the machines – but many have been sold to the layman and unfortunately are often used to the detriment, rather than advantage, of the patient. This book is an attempt to explain in relatively simple terms the construction of the musculoskeletal system, the effects on that system of injury and the repair processes of the system along with a description of the methods of aiding the repair, whether this be by the simple applications of heat, cold and massage or with sophisticated machines.

It is very important to realise that there can be no exact criteria as to treatment times or dosage – each case must be judged on individual circumstances. It is also important to recognise that no one machine can be adapted to fulfil all requirements; each has a specific effect. The purpose of the machines is to enhance the healing abilities of the body, minimise secondary trauma and restore full function to the injured area.

Some of the machines, by stimulation of specific cells, may induce an earlier start to the natural repair processes of the body, but the claim that machines accelerate healing has yet to be proven.

The body systems

Trying to visualise the complexity of a living being is as daunting as trying to comprehend space. A grasp of essentials is, however, necessary in order to understand the problems associated with injury.

Both horse and rider are constructed from similar components or systems. The basic unit of life is the cell, and these cells bond together and form differing systems of the body.

System		Function
Skeletal system	– bones	
Joints	– articulation	Locomotor
Muscles	– movement	
Respiratory system	– lungs	Oxygen/gas interchange
Vascular system	– heart/veins/arteries	Conveyance
Lymphatic system	– glands	Filter system
		Disease defence
Nervous system	– brain/spinal cord/nerves	Central control of all systems
		Sensation recording
		Message carriers
Digestive system	– stomach/intestine	Food uptake for energy
		Waste disposal
Urinary system	– bladder/kidneys	Liquid filtration
Reproductive system		

Bones

Bones are of differing designs, their shape and size varying with their functional requirements. Bone is the hardest tissue in the body with the exception of the teeth. It provides the framework, the support of the body, and protects certain internal organs. It gives attachments for muscles and tendons as well as constituting the levers the muscles move. The structure of bone allows great strength. It is subjected to compression, tension, twisting and bending strains, and is able to withstand these stresses by virtue of a certain amount of elasticity.

Long bones, or limb bones, have a central cavity, a factory producing certain cells. At each end of a long bone, before maturity, is an *epiphyseal plate*. This is a cartilage-type plate from which the long or limb bones grow. At maturity this plate has completed its function and turns into exactly the same structure as its parent bone. The bones of the skull, the ribs and the shoulder blades are known as *flat bones*. *Sesamoid bones* are small rounded masses found in certain tendons at points of friction. The largest of these sesamoid bones is the *patella*, located on the front of the knee in man and on the front of the stifle in the horse. All bones are covered by an outer skin or *periosteum*, this giving support to the blood vessels that feed the bone and also allowing for the attachment of the fibres of muscles, tendons, ligaments and the capsules of joints.

Joints

Joints are the meeting places between bones. Some meeting places, like those of the differing bones of the skull, have no movement (*articulation*) between them. Another example is found in the pelvis at the *sacroiliac joints*. The majority of joints, however, are *synovial joints* (Fig. 1) and allow for free movement between the bone ends. In this type of joint the ends of the bones are covered with a cartilage, *hyaline cartilage*. The cartilage is smooth and has a very low coefficient of friction, ensuring a slippery surface that allows for easy movement. Cartilage acts in part as a shock absorber and assists, in a small way, in the lubrication of the joint.

Joints are enveloped by a sleeve or *capsular ligament*. The cells on the inner surface of this tissue produce *synovial fluid*, or joint oil. Working alone, the capsule would be unable to support and restrain the movement between the opposing bones ends, and support is assisted by *ligaments*.

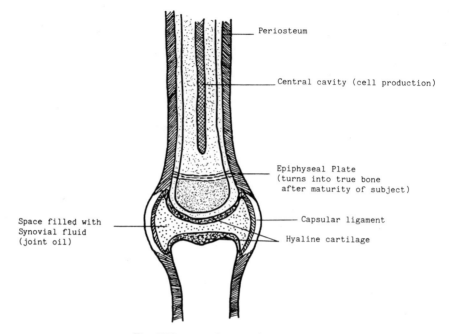

Fig. 1 Diagram of a synovial joint.

Ligaments

Ligaments are composed of strong tissue. They are usually arranged in flat bands, the bands running across the joint, outside the capsule, and arranged in such a way as to give maximal support for the functions of that particular joint. Movement outside normal range sprains ligaments. Unlike muscle, they do not have an elastic quality; they merely allow for some adaptation to stretch forces. Ligaments have an inadequate blood (*vascular*) supply but are rich in sensory nerve. Involved in over-stretch, they give rise to immediate pain which can be severe. They are slow to heal.

Muscle

The type of muscle that moves one bone upon another and produces the movement required for activity is known as *skeletal muscle*. It is of a differing construction from the muscle that drives the heart, *cardiac muscle*, and also differs from the muscle that forms the hollow internal organs, the *bladder*, the *bowels*, the *intestines* and the *blood vessels*.

Composed of a series of components or muscle *spindles*, skeletal muscles are highly elastic. Controlled by *motor nerves*, they shorten, or *contract*, as the result of a signal transmitted via a nerve.

In any one muscle only a proportion of the total mass is working at any one time.

Muscles are described as starting or arising (*origin*), from an area proximal (*proximal* – a point nearer to the centre of the body) to their ending (*insertion*) in an area distal (*distal* – a point further from the centre of the body) to their origin. They are attached to the *periosteum* and underlying bone rather as seaweed is attached to a rock.

Some muscles end in *tendons*.

Tendons

Tendons (Fig. 2) have the ability to sustain enormous loads due to a high tensile strength. Their fibres are not elastic as are the fibres of their parent muscle, but at rest they exhibit a crimp-like appearance. When the tendon is under stress this crimp, in part, disappears, returning only when the stretch force is removed. The blood, or vascular, supply to a tendon must be considered inadequate to cope with the stresses and strains imposed by the competition requirements of today.

Functionally, tendons have the ability to concentrate the pull of their parent muscle upon a small area. In the horse they also assist in the support of joints – for example, aiding the suspensory ligament in the support of the fetlock. Man has no structure comparable to the deep and superficial digital flexor tendons found in the lower limbs of large animals, the nearest human equivalent being the *Achilles*, or heel, tendon.

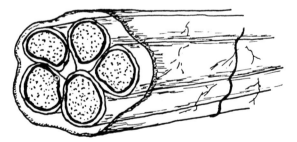

Fig. 2 Diagram of a tendon in cross section. The structure resembles a parachute cord.

Respiratory system

The respiratory system starts in the nasal passages, which lead into a rigid tube called the *larynx*; the larynx becomes the windpipe or *trachea*. Passing into the chest cavity, it divides into two main branches known as *bronchi*. The sub-division of the bronchi into masses of tiny tubes, each ending in a small air sac – the *alveolus sacs* – forms the *lung tissue*. The walls of the air sacs support a plexus of blood vessels; it is through the walls of the air sacs that the uptake, by the blood, of the oxygen required and the dumping of the carbon-dioxide waste not required takes place. Oxygen is a vital requirement for the correct working of the body systems. The amount of oxygen in the lung tissue, available for collection, is dependent on the rate (speed) and depth (expansion of chest) of breathing, or *respiration*.

The speed at which the oxygen passes to the working areas is dependent on the rate and strength of the heartbeats. Thus the respiratory and circulatory systems are inextricably linked.

The heart

The heart is a large muscular organ with four chambers, its function being to propel blood through the body by alternate contraction and relaxation. A specialist muscle, it is supplied with a circulatory system of its own, the *coronary system*, and a highly complex nervous system. This nervous system automatically controls the rate and depth of heart beat; that is, the individual cannot control voluntarily the heart performance. The organ responds rapidly to changes within the body, for example, a sudden *adrenaline* release accelerates the heart rate.

The beat rate of the heart in the resting horse is normally 30 to 40 beats per minute. In the human, the beat ranges between the low 60s and the middle 80s. (The significance of heart rate and its return to normal in exercise will be discussed later.)

Circulation

The circulatory, or *vascular*, system forms the transport mechanism of the body and can be related to a conveyor belt. It is a closed-circuit system, with the flow of blood achieved by the pumping action of the heart. Blood is a fluid in which are suspended many differing types of cell: some carry oxygen, some nutrients, while some remove waste products. The mechanism of clotting and stopping blood loss after injury is initiated by other types of cells suspended in the blood fluid.

Circulatory flow is of the greatest importance after injury, and circulation can be regarded as the transport system bringing the healing agents to, and removing the waste and debris from, the injured area.

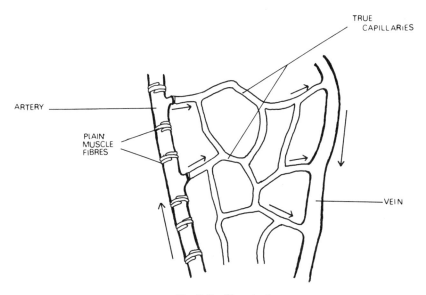

Fig. 3 Capillary bed.

Blood leaves the heart and is forced through the *arteries*. The arteries break down from large-diameter tubes to the tiny little vessels of the *capillary bed* (Fig. 3). In the capillary bed, the vital exchanges between the tissues and the blood take place. The capillaries have very thin walls, described as *semi-permeable*. These walls are highly selective and determine the passage of materials to and from the surrounding tissue.

As the arterial system ended in the capillary bed, so does the *venous system* arise. The vessels regroup and form tiny *veins* which, in their turn, branch and form the large veins of the circulatory system.

Blood in the *arteries*, known as *arterial blood*, is that carrying nutrients and oxygen to the tissues. Blood in the *veins*, *venous blood*, transports waste, passing through various cleansing organs as it goes. Then, via the heart, it returns to the lungs, ready to give up carbon dioxide and collect the next load of oxygen.

The return of venous blood is greatly assisted by muscle contracture. Arteries have strong muscular walls and the effect of the heartbeat is to push blood through them. There is no suction method to draw the venous blood back to the heart but the very fact that more arterial blood travels forward with each heartbeat does create a pressure effect. To cope with the return of blood via the veins, the vessels are supplied with small valves. These cup-like valves fill, and close off sections of vein between each heartbeat, ensuring a one-way flow. When subjected to pressure by contracting vessels, the veins, whose walls are less muscular than those of the arteries, are compressed, allowing blood to be squeezed from section to section. The venous system is assisted by the *lymphatic system.*

Lymphatic system

Lymph vessels are similar in structure to veins, containing valves and having thin walls. The system functions in part as a back-up mechanism to the venous circulation, assisting by moving excess fluid, but its most important function is that of the filtering and destruction of harmful substances. Throughout the system are situated clusters of glands known as *lymph glands.* They serve as one of the barriers to infection by producing antibodies and specialist cells called *lympho-cytes.* Lymphocytes act as scavengers.

Another important function of the circulatory system is the control of body temperature. A body that is too cold cannot function. The superficial vessels narrow or contract, centralizing the blood and ensuring the maintenance of the correct temperature of the vital organs such as the brain, the heart and the lungs. Conversely, to maintain correct temperature should the body become overheated, the surface vessels dilate and in this way are able to lose heat through the skin.

Nervous system

The nervous system provides the communication network and can be regarded as a series of highly complex and interlinking computers, the centralised computer being the *brain.* The brain is composed of specialist nervous tissue.

Some of the functions of the body can be controlled by conscious thought. Other functions are not controlled, and continue as an automatic occurrence due to the computer-like behaviour of central nervous tissue.

The brain has an extension known as the *spinal cord.* This extension is well protected by the bones comprising the *vertebral column,* the brain itself being protected by the bones of the *skull.*

At each intersection between the *vertebral bodies* (bones of the spine), a pair of nerves emerge. These nerves consist of hundreds of tiny filaments and in cross-section, under a microscope, would resemble a cut main telephone wire. The nerves divide and sub-divide within the body, each nerve protected by an outer sheath, or *axon,* and each branch preparing for a specific function.

Nerves end in differing tissue and, according to their predetermined functions, take messages to an area, carry messages from an area, and record all manner of information.

Nervous tissue is very susceptible to pressure. If continuous pressure is applied, nerves may cease to be able to pass messages, or *conduct*. This may leave an area of the body without sensation and/or the muscles in that area may have an ineffective communication relay. Known as an *impaired nerve supply*, this will cause a muscle to waste, or *atrophy*.

The skeleton

The bony skeleton (Figs 4 and 5) serves as a framework for other body tissues to build upon, and also in part as a protection for some of the vital organs. The skull houses the brain, the central vital computer composed of specialist-type nerve tissue, *central nervous tissue*. An extension of the brain, ably protected by the bones of the back or vertebral column, is known as the *spinal cord*. (Damage to the tissue of the brain or the spinal cord is final, no repair or recovery being possible. Dependent on the level of accident, loss of a particular function or series of functions occurs.) The first set of bones of the vertebral column are the neck bones (*cervical vertebrae*). Movements in the cervical area of the horse are up and down and from side to side.

In the human there is more rotation between the first two cervical vertebrae and the skull than in the horse. The human can also move up (extension) and down (forward flexion), and from side to side. The cervical vertebrae join to the chest, or *thoracic* area. From the bones of the *thoracic vertebrae* arise the *ribs*, curving forward, shaped rather like bucket handles and meeting the breast bone, or *sternum*, at the front and forming the bony chest cage. This cage is partitioned by the *diaphragm*, a large sheet of muscle, its function being to aid breathing.

Rotation is present in the human thorax, with side bending and some forward and backward bending. There are muscle arrangements which produce these movements. The four-point balance of the horse and the muscle arrangement allow movement to occur both up (*dorsiflex*) and down (*ventroflexion*) and from side to side, but there is no muscle arrangement which creates these movements: they occur only because the vertebral column is a jointed structure.

The lungs lie in the upper (human) or forward (horse) compartment of the thoracic cage, with the heart cushioned between them. Below (human) or behind (horse) the diaphragm are the abdominal contents.

The last thoracic vertebra joins the first *lumbar vertebra*. The

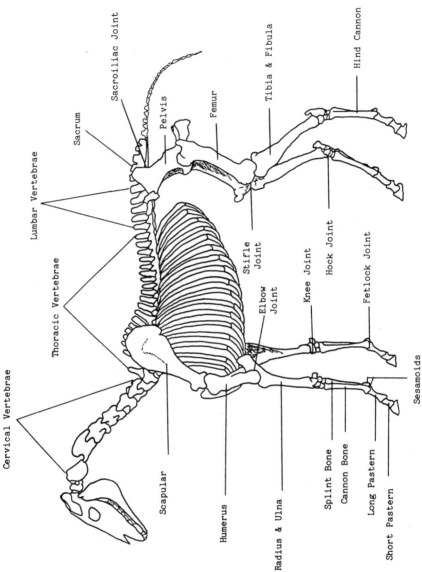

Fig. 4 The horse's skeleton.

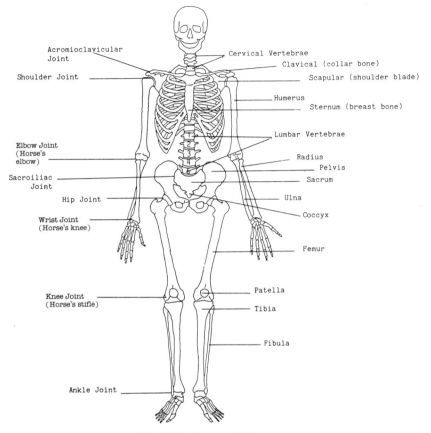

Fig. 5 The human skeleton.

lumbar vertebrae form the low back (human) or loins (horse). The vertebrae bridge the gap between the chest, or thoracic cage, and the *pelvis*, the last lumbar vertebra joining a triangular block of fused bone, the *sacrum*, which ends in the small bones of the tai, or *coccyx*.

The two halves of the pelvis (*pelvic bones*) curve round and meet the triangle of fused bone, the sacrum, at the *sacroiliac joints*, so named because the upper part of the bone of the pelvis is called the *ilium*. The sacroiliac joint has no muscular control and, while termed a joint, is merely the meeting place of two bones. It appears to act as a type of primitive shock absorber.

Hindlimb

The hindlimbs of the horse and lower limbs of the human are locked to the pelvic girdle through two sockets: the *acetabulum*, two depressions shaped like deep saucers, into which fit the ball-like heads of the upper bone of the limb, the *femur*, or thigh bone (the strongest bone of the body in both horse and human). Below this bone, any similarity between human and horse ceases.

The thigh of the human ends at the knee; the two bones below, the *tibia* and the *fibula*, lock at their base to form and grip the first bone of the foot, the *talus*, and form the ankle joint. The bones of the human foot are arranged and shaped in a series of of arches and levers, designed for forward and upward propulsion and also to absorb and dissipate the shock of meeting the ground. In front of the knee of the human is a sesamoid bone, the *patella*, encased within the tendonous ends of the large muscles that lie on the front of the thigh, the *quadriceps*. Sesamoid bones are often present on either side of the first joint of the big toe in the human.

Equivalent to the human knee in the horse is the *stifle*. From there, the tibia and fibula fuse at their *distal*, or lower, end, angle backwards and end at the hock. The horse stands on a single central bone, the *cannon*, with two accessory bones, the *splint bones*, lying on either side but serving no structural function. The cannon bones angle slightly forward, meeting the *long pastern* at the fetlock joint; behind this joint there are two sesamoid bones, the *proximal sesamoids*. The first *phalanx*, or long pastern, articulates at its distal end with the second *phalanx*, or short pastern, in its turn balanced on the *pedal* or *coffin* bone.

Forelimb

In the human, the arm is hung from a yoke-like structure consisting of the shoulder blade, or *scapula* (lying on the back of the chest), and attached to the collar bone, or *clavicle* (lying on the front of the chest). The collar bone, in its turn, is attached to the *sternum*, the central front bone of the thoracic (chest) cage. There is a depression on the scapula which allows movement of the head of the upper bone of the arm, the *humerus*.

The forearm of the human consists of two bones, the *radius* and the *ulna*. Movement at the elbow joint is in two plains, bending (flexion) and straightening (extension). The ability of the human to turn the palm of the hand in two directions occurs between the radius and the ulna, at a joint below the elbow joint known as the *radio-ulna joint*. The distal end of the radius and ulna articulate with the small bones of the wrist, which in their turn articulate with the bones in the hands and fingers.

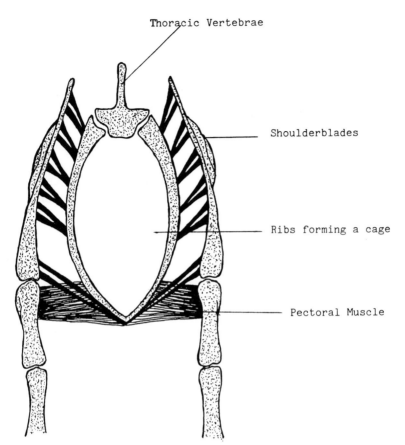

Thoracic Vertebrae

Shoulderblades

Ribs forming a cage

Pectoral Muscle

Fig. 6 Diagram to demonstrate the suspension structure of the forehand of the horse.

In the horse, the forelimb supports two-thirds of the animal's body weight. There are no collar bones; the arrangement of the shoulder blades (*scapulae*), ligaments and muscles enable the weight to be slung, as in a cradle, between the two forelimbs (Fig. 6). The humerus angles backwards from the distal end of the shoulder blade, and meets a fused radius and ulna (bones of the upper limb) at the horse's elbow. The knee of the horse corresponds to the human wrist; below the knee, the bone arrangement is exactly similar to that of the hindlimb.

Skeletal muscle

As discussed, the bony skeleton not only provides the frame or structural base for the attachment of skeletal muscle, i.e. those muscles that produce movement, but also relies on the skeletal muscle groups for support. Ligaments alone cannot hold up the skeleton: they rely on a partnership with the muscles.

The sites of attachment, the arrangements of the groups, the angle of lie of the fibres, and the direction of pull that occurs when muscles shorten or contract determine all movement sequences.

Passing over joints, muscles assist in the stability of the joint as well as creating movement. In some cases, fibres from the muscle blend with the fibres of the joint capsule. This combination provides protection, for, should the joint become forced towards a movement range beyond its anatomical normal, the excessive tension on the joint capsule is moderated by contraction of the overlying muscle fibres.

No one muscle works on its own: all movement is a group effort. For movement to occur, many activities take place; vast quantities of information are collected, recorded and analysed by the nervous system in a manner that can be likened to the interaction of banks of computers all interlinking, all dependent one upon the other and, in the case of the body, controlled by certain centres in the brain.

A microscopic proportion of the activities of the body are conscious. The vast majority are reflex; that is, they occur without conscious effort or thought.

Muscles can only produce effective, efficient movement patterns if they are in balance; that is, the strength of one group is complimentary to its partner groups. Both sides of the body must work in harmony and there must be equal power between left and right.

Injury, no matter if it is to bone, joint, ligament, tendon, nerve or to a muscle or group of muscles, causes degeneration and impaired function of the muscles injured or that control the section of the body injured.

This muscle degeneration or atrophy occurs for any one of a number of reasons, among them:

- *Disuse atrophy*: due to pain, the area is not used.
- *Loss of nerve conduction*: a muscle with no communication system, unable to relay or receive messages, atrophies rapidly.
- *Destruction of the muscle structure*: crushing, bruising, tearing or the presence of chemical toxins (secondary to cellular damage) causes muscle tissue to deteriorate.
- *Ischaemia*: loss of blood supply due to disruption of circulatory flow.
- *Excessive exercise*: due to lack of fuel, muscle tissue breaks down.

Some muscles appear to degenerate, or waste, faster than others –

muscles without a nerve supply or with an impaired nerve supply lose functional ability immediately. The apparent reduction in bulk, when contrasted with the uninjured opposite muscle, can be startlingly visible within a few days. Palpation also reveals reduction in bulk.

As the injury recovers so will muscle begin to regenerate, whether treated or not, *but* unless treated it is very unlikely to regain the strength and ability enjoyed prior to injury. As activity is resumed, the strong muscles, under exercise pressure, get stronger, they do not sit around and wait for the weak muscle to regain its original strength, allowing balanced movement patterns. This factor is the main reason for the recurrence of the original problem at a later date and/or the inability of the animal to achieve the performance levels enjoyed before injury.

Electrical stimulation of muscle followed by an exercise pattern designed to re-educate the weak areas is the surest way to regain full potential.

Reflex movement patterns

All movement patterns occur as a result of learning. The baby falls endlessly while learning to walk; the foal learns faster, but is hesitant and uncontrolled in early life. Gradually, *reflex* patterns are established; that is, movement sequences occur as an automatic response to a set of circumstances, with the brain, via the nervous system, activating the necessary computer responses.

In the case of the ridden horse, most responses occur as the result of signals given by the rider. Injury and subsequent lay off may cause these previously automatic responses to be lost – there is a computer failure. Inability of the rider to appreciate this causes many problems, the rider expecting the horse to perform to command to the exact standard that had been achieved at the time of injury.

Start slowly and re-educate to avoid disappointment.

2   Injury – Effects and Repair

The effects of injury

Bone damage

Damage to bone equals loss of support in the framework/leverage system. Broken bones are known as *fractured bones*. There are many different types of fracture: complete fractures are a crack or break with the line of the break passing through the bone in its entirety; bones may be broken in one or more places, they may be crushed, or just cracked. They are slow to heal but, provided the ends are approximated – that is, opposite each other – and movement between the bone ends or between the bone particles/pieces is eliminated, healing will occur.

Fractures are best diagnosed by X-ray. X-ray is comparatively easy throughout the human skeletal system, but other than in the limbs of the horse a highly sophisticated X-ray apparatus, not readily available, is required because of the depth of tissue.

Repair phases of the recovery of bone are similar to those of soft tissue. In the case of bone, the end result is probably the most perfect for similarity of structure. Complete fractures usually need to be immobilised for good repair. In a weight-bearing limb this is almost impossible in the horse but, with the expansion of veterinary orthopaedic surgery, the use of pins, plates and screws, a great number of horses, who a decade ago would have been put down, can now be saved.

Cracks can be successfully treated without the need for the limb to be immobilised. Of these, the most common condition is that of sore shins. Localised stresses (an occupational hazard of athletic bone) causes minute cracks in the cannon bone. Early X-ray is usually normal but later X-ray may show *callus* formation where the tiny cracks are trying to heal. Callus is new bone and shows only on X-ray. In American terminology, this condition is termed *bucked shins*.

Early lameness denoting this condition may be minimal, but the pain may suddenly rise to a crescendo, with lameness and hypersensitivity to touch. A history of pain and tenderness should lead to at least three weeks of reduced activity, accompanied by treatment from an appropriate machine. Ignored, stress fractures continue to give trouble and in some cases a spontaneous complete fracture occurs.

Damage to the periosteum

The periosteum is the outer covering or the outer skin of the bones. Muscles, ligaments and tendons are contiguous with the periosteum at their origins and insertions. Tears, pulls or knocks cause rupture of small blood vessels, with consequent bleeding. This bleeding is an irritant to the bone and, in order to protect itself, new bone grows, forming small ridges or lumps. These may interfere with normal function if adjacent to a joint or tendon. Bleeding between the bone and periosteum also causes severe pain.

Damage to the epiphyseal plates

Long bones, or limb bones, grow from specialist-type plates called *epiphyseal plates*. The long bones of the horse are not fully grown (*ossified*) before the age of two; in some bones – for example, the ulna – the epiphyseal plate is present until the animal is at least three years old. Under certain stress conditions and with over-training, these plates become irritated and inflamed; the condition is termed *epiphysitis* – that is, inflammation of the epiphyseal plate.

Damage to bursæ

Bursæ are small sacs of fluid, built in to various points of the body in areas of possible friction. Their function is to stop bone rubbing and so damaging the under surface of an overlying muscle. Bursæ can become inflamed. When this occurs, they swell and cause severe pain and restricted movement.

Damage to joints

The correct terminology for joint damage is *arthritis* (arth = joint, itis = inflammation). An inflamed joint is an *arthritic joint*. Until the word arthritis has a descriptive adjective attached it does not necessarily mean there will be irreversible joint changes. An irreversible joint change termed *osteo-arthritic* is where the bone ends forming the joint have grown irregularities round the circumference, impeding joint movement.

Joints are *sprained* being put through a range of motion greater than they were anatomically designed to perform. This excessive movement may damage surrounding muscle tissue and also the supporting ligaments.

Damage to ligament

Ligaments support joints. Over-stretched ligaments therefore lead to loss of stability in the joint. In the case of the *suspensory ligament*, stability is lost at the fetlock joint and below.

Damage to interosseous ligaments

These ligaments lie between two adjacent bones (inter = between, osseous = bone); for example, between the splint and the cannon bone. Tears of an interosseous ligament cause pain in the first instance and laying down of new bone in the second; dependent on the position of the new growth, interference with normal function may occur. Some degree of pain is usually present in the early active stage of injury.

Damage to muscle

Muscle damage causes ineffective, incorrect and unbalanced movement patterns. Weakness will occur as a result of torn fibres. Muscle atrophy (loss of muscle tissue) occurs as a result of disuse and/or loss of communication due to damage to motor nerves.

Damage to tendon

Damage to a tendon occurs in the most part due to over-stretch, associated with a tired or weak parent muscle. There is loss of full effective function in the limb. A structural weakness occurs in the affected limb, which may be permanent. The parent muscle also shows impaired functional weakness.

Tendon tissue has, as yet, not been simulated in a manner that has caused the original type fibre to reform after injury.

Damage to nerve

Pressure upon or severance of nerves equals loss of communication. Dependent upon the type of nerve tissue involved, there may be loss of skin sensation, or loss of appreciation of position in space of a limb or part of a limb. Muscles waste, or *atrophy*, if their motor nerve is damaged.

All functions are dependent on a normal nerve supply. Should damage be to the specialist nerve tissue of the brain or spinal cord, the damage is final and recovery does not occur. Damage to nerve tissue outside the brain and spinal cord is not always final.

Injury and repair

Injury is a catastrophe. No matter which structure is the prime sight, all the body systems are affected to a greater or lesser degree. The ancient Chinese description of the need for the perfect balance between the systems is very apt, for without balance within the musculoskeletal and associated systems, athletic ability is seriously impaired. Contrary to the popular belief that 'rest is the only cure' and/or 'time is the only healer', up-to-date knowledge derived from experimental work on tissue in the laboratories of the world shows that controlled early activity is beneficial.

The application of modern technology in the shape of machines enhances and assists the body's rebuilding mechanisms, provided that the correct machine is used at the correct time and that early treatment is followed by graded exercise.

To try to imagine what happens when injury occurs. Envisage a bomb falling on a city and the consequent devastation: heaps of debris, leakage of liquids, escape of gases, disruption of communication – all leading to loss of function of the area. Rebuilding the area needs a carefully prepared plan of campaign if the city is to be restored to its original state. In living tissue, *pain* is an added complication, producing many side effects and hindering, by invoking muscle spasm, circulatory flow to the area and thus complicating the repair process. If, after injury, reparation is rushed, there may be loss of performance ability, leading to lack of confidence in both horse and rider – particularly when performing a task similar to that from which the injury resulted.

As with a bomb a plan of campaign for rehabilitation is necessary. The plan will vary, depending on the severity of the injury and the response of the individual to the treatments given. There can be no hard and fast rules laid down, as is possible when reconstructing a building.

The reaction of the body tissues, whatever the cause of the injury, is immediate and similar: to rebuild. Reparative measures far in excess of those required are activated and, given the best possible conditions, damaged tissue will do its best to reproduce to its original state.

Healing of the tissues is divided into three phases which overlap: the first, named *inflammation*; the second, *proliferation*; and the third, *remodelling*.

Inflammation

At the site of injury, the structure involved has broken down. Small blood vessels rupture, blood escapes into the area of damage, and fluids and cells leak from tissue spaces adjacent to the broken structures. Tissue around the site may also be stretched or torn. Dependent on the severity of the injury, the nerve pathways involved may cease to conduct.

Obvious signs at this phase are swelling, warmth, loss of full function and pain, the latter exhibited both on pressure and during attempted movement. Pain is caused by the presence of toxic substances in the area of sensory nerve endings and/or increased pressure on pain-recording nerve endings.

The irritant chemicals, the result of cell destruction, and the free blood in the tissue act as a stimulant for the arrival of an excess of fluids bearing cells. Some of the fluids seeping through vessel walls may damage normal tissue surrounding the actual site of injury.

Other specialist cells migrate rapidly to the area of damage and begin the task of clearing away *debris*, or the dead tissue. The migrating cells continue to irritate surrounding tissues, this irritation acting as a stimulant to ensure the continuous flow of blood to the site. The problem then arising and which is due to the immobility of the local tissues (the result of the pain and swelling or because immobilisation is called for) is that the venous return, dependent as it is on muscle contraction, is impaired. The area becomes engorged; the lack of rapid clearance of these excess fluids and cells leads to the formation of a *haematoma*.

Should the fluids and cells not be reabsorbed from the surrounding area, sections of overlying tissue become adherent, one to the other. *Adhesions* restrict movement; worse still, when stretched they break down and the entire healing process has to recommence in an area adjacent to, but not involved in, the original incident.

Proliferation

At the end of approximately a week following injury, new blood vessels have started growing throughout the area, only primitive at the early stages but capable of transporting blood. The less solid the haematoma, the more able are these new vessels to work their way through the tissue. Remember the circulation is the conveyor belt, taking away the damaged and destroyed tissue and bringing in the repair materials. Building cells arrive via the new blood vessels and begin to lay down rope-like fibres of the tissue from which all body tissues are constructed – *collagen* – and a *scar* is formed. Seen under a microscope, approximately 10 days after injury, the tissues often look like a badly darned sock. Once the body computers are satisfied that the gap between the broken ends has been bridged by the *scar*, remodelling begins.

Remodelling

Remodelling is the final stage of repair and takes many months. There are no set times that can be applied to the process. Tissue will always try to reproduce itself after injury in a state as near to the original as possible. During this phase, small fibres attempt to push through the scar.

Remodelling is more successful in some tissues than in others. Bone produces the most perfect result. Muscle fibres remodel well if the scar in their midst is kept soft and mobile.

Central nervous tissue never recovers its original state, the scars that form in the area of damage preventing communication from the brain to the areas below the level of the injury. This is hard to comprehend and deserves explanation.

Peripheral nervous tissue should be visualised as a domestic ring-main system, the nerves conducting messages of all types along their fibres in a manner similar to the passage of electricity along the domestic cables in your house. The central core of the nerve is insulated, just as the electrical wires are, by an outer covering or sheath. Undue pressure on the sheath prevents the passage of the electrical current, and the nerve ceases to pass messages until the pressure is removed. Should the nerve be severed, provided the two cut ends are in touch with each other, it will, though temporarily unable to pass messages, in time repair itself and regain function.

Central nervous tissue, comprising the brain and spinal cord, is composed of a very much more highly sophisticated tissue serving both as a generating centre and a switchboard. The protection given this tissue by the skull and the bony canal of the vertebral column should render adequate protection from injury; no reparative processes are available.

Confusion often arises when, after an accident, the term 'broken back' is used. A broken bone in the back repairs, given time. Provided the spinal cord is not involved, full functional recovery is possible. Involve the spinal cord in such a manner that it is cut, and the picture becomes very serious: the damaged area ceases to pass messages, and there is no communication between the central switch board, the generating centre and the areas of the body below the area of damage. A broken neck involving the spinal cord results in total paralysis below the level of the break; a broken back involving the spinal cord results in total paralysis below the level of the break – for example, loss of the use of both legs.

Doctors working in America are trying to develop an implant that can be inserted surgically at the level of the break in the spinal cord and will allow the electrical currents from the brain to flow unimpeded across the gap, thus allowing full functional activity below the level of damage to be regained.

Possible causes of injury

Human athletic injuries occur as a result of (a) lack of fitness; (b) poor conformation; (c) poor equipment; (d) poor technique; (e) accident. Of these causes, accident forms the smallest number of incidents, the accident often occuring as a result of (a), (b), (c) or (d).

The above causes are all applicable to the horse, but to them must be added the rider, the rider's weight, and the rider's ability and *fitness*.

Lack of fitness

Fitness and *preparation* for the task or tasks the horse will eventually be required to perform must go hand in hand. A horse is born with a brain which soon after birth learns to react to external stimuli. Training a horse involves increasing the ability of the animal to respond and react to a series of new stimuli invoked by the rider, many of which his natural living conditions would never demand. Some horses learn fast, some slowly; their apparent mistakes are often a result of their being asked to perform a task to which they have not previously been exposed, despite the fact that they may be physically fit. Fitness is not just the ability to gallop a mile and not be exhausted: it is the ability to gallop a mile balanced, on uneven ground, even crossing a series of obstacles en route in a balanced, controlled way, carrying a mobile weight – the rider. No mean task.

Good conformation, fitness for the task, a sound basic training and the rider's ability to help when needed – and leave well alone when not – are the basic essentials for the avoidance of injury.

Poor conformation

Horses come in many shapes and sizes. Down the ages, cross and line breeding have endeavoured to produce the best possible shape for the task the particular breed is to perform. Amongst other things, an 'eye for a horse' is the ability to look at an animal and decide if its overall conformation is suitable for the discipline for which it will be trained. The old saying 'you cannot make a silk purse out of a sow's ear' along with 'never buy trouble, it comes soon enough' could well be borne in mind when considering the purchase of an animal. Conformation weaknesses nearly always cause trouble when an animal is pressed to its limit.

Limbs should be of sufficient strength to carry the frame. Long cannon bones and a short forearm are more susceptible to breakdown than short cannon bones and a long forearm. The longer the cannon, the greater the length of and therefore stress on the tendons.

A well-developed second thigh, or gaskin, is essential for the support of the hock. Hocks are the focal point for manoeuvrability when a horse endeavours to leave the ground. Good hocks are a must: curbs, spavins and thoroughpins all arise from weak hocks.

Much more could be said about conformation, but it should be taken into account after injury and corrective measures taken to try to remove any underlying problem. Remember, injury in one area may well have occurred because of a problem in another area. Recent papers have shown that some horses, said by their owners to have 'backs', were suffering from a variety of limb problems which caused them to work out of balance. The back condition was secondary – treatment of the limb problem cured the back!

Poor equipment

A horse tries to first avoid and then evade pain, and in doing so will form bad habits which are difficult to break. Incorrect bitting, *badly fitting saddles*, and overtight boots or bandages are all contributory factors in the pattern of eventual injury.

Poor technique

The inexperience or inability of the rider to teach the horse results in poor technique. Technique is of particular importance when the horse leaves the ground. Basic schooling is an essential in the avoidance of injury, whatever the eventual discipline of the horse.

Accidents caused by the horse alone are rare; accidents usually involve rider mistakes or unexpected external events.

The greatest cause of self-imposed accident leading to injury is a horse getting cast. He is not clever enough to judge the distance between himself and the box wall. As he rolls over, he cannot complete the roll, his centre of gravity being too close to the wall, and he gets stuck. If the wall has no purchase points, the upper hind leg, trying to push the body away from the wall, slides upward in an uncontrolled manner, often causing severe damage in the hip and pelvic area. Anti-cast strips are well worth fitting to the interior walls of loose boxes.

A second cause of self-imposed stable injury is insufficient bedding, particularly on a floor without ridges. As the horse rises after lying down, the metal shoe, in contact with the floor, slides across the slippery base, causing injury in the pelvic area. Any readers who have worn steel heel clips on their shoes must at some time have lost their footing on a slippery surface.

All-weather surfaces and gallops

Many types of all-weather surfaces are available, and all present different problems: none as yet is a substitute for old turf, with its natural spring to cushion impact, and porous soil beneath rather than 'dead' ground.

To be hypercritical, it could be said these new surfaces have increased rather than lessened problems.

The greatest difficulty is to maintain an even, sound, surface. Think of the experience of running on firm sand – suddenly the surface changes and you sink in for a few strides; your back is jarred, your stride changes, and if you were running at speed you stumble and may even fall.

The effect on a horse may not be quite as dramatic, but the potential for injury is there and many small injuries do occur – often, as previously described, without obvious clinical signs.

A spate of small injuries in a yard, after work on an all-weather surface, should alert trainers to the possibility of a piece of false ground, and steps should be taken to discover and remedy the fault.

All-weather surfaces on an uphill slope are notorious for causing sore backs in two-year-olds. Immature and often off the bridle, they leave a hind leg behind, with consequent muscle and ligament problems – problems that are all too often increased when they roll due to discomfort and get cast after exercise.

Tooth problems as a cause of injury

Problems within the horse's mouth are often neglected. Regular dental checks should be as much a part of good health management as regular shoeing. Unfortunately, the horse dentist is a rare bird. It is impossible to examine the back teeth, the cause of most troubles, effectively without a gag (see Plate 1). As the lower jaw is narrower than the upper, the back teeth of the horse do not meet in perfect alignment. The chew action is a cross sweep, grinding one row of teeth across the other. Gradually, sharp edges are created on the outer edges of the back teeth of the upper jaw; unnoticed, they may cut the insides of the cheeks. In the lower jaw these edges form on the inner side of the teeth, rubbing against the tongue, often making it sore and sometimes causing small ulcers. The edges, often razor sharp, must be filed to round them off. This is skilled work, as although ivory is a very durable substance it is possible to damage teeth while filing them.

Dental cavities are rare, but gum infections cause abscesses involving teeth, and these give rise to pain. Fractures of teeth occur, the animal mistakenly picking up and chewing on a hard object, or being 'caught in the mouth', the result of incorrect bitting and/or handling of the bit by the rider. The pain experienced must be similar to that felt by the human when biting on an unexpected solid object whilst chewing, as the horse's tooth has a nerve supply similar to the human's.

A horse with a painful mouth will do his best to evade pain, resisting and fighting against contact with the bit. In doing so, his head position will change and the horse will become 'out of balance'; remember how important the head position is for the support of the back.

Pain in the mouth affecting the correct chewing action will effect nutrition. Incorrectly chewed food is not digested and absorbed as it should be; if you think saving on dentistry is an economy, consider the rise in your food bills as you endeavour to 'feed up' your 'poor' horse.

Check mouths on a regular basis: six months is the maximum time that should elapse between dental checks. In addition, two-year-olds should be checked to see if the outer 'shells' of their back teeth are

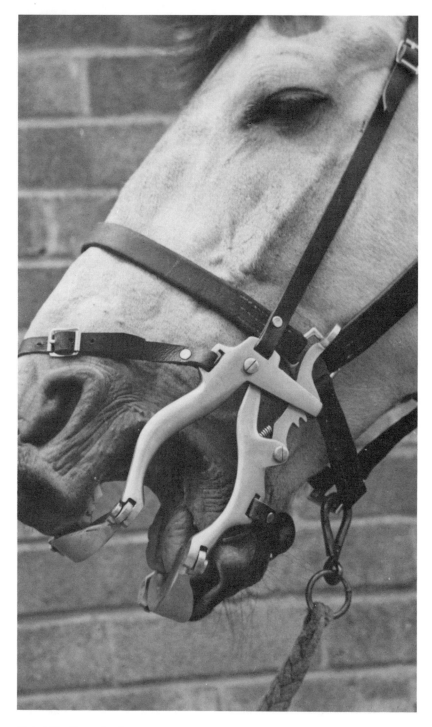

Plate 1 Tooth gag in place.

loose and have not shed naturally. Wolf teeth need to be removed when they are fully through the gum.

In a young horse with a particularly sensitive mouth, a rubber bit may be advisable; but whatever type of bit is used, it must fit. All horses have different shaped mouths and what fits one may not fit another. Think how you feel if the dentist takes an impression and misjudges the size of your mouth, over-filling it with the impression mould.

A horse unhappy in the mouth will not give of his best, and will learn both bad habits and an incorrect way of going. These factors may eventually contribute to some form of musculoskeletal injury.

The foot and shoe as a possible cause of injury

Long gaps between shoeing, a horse turned out with untrimmed feet – both are false economies. No foot, no horse: a good foot is one of the determining factors in the ability of the animal to stay sound and perform well.

The direction of hoof growth is downward and forward. If the toe is allowed to grow too long and the heels are too short, the critical angle of the pastern is changed. Damage to the flexor tendons may occur due to the increased strain. The angle of the hoof to the ground should be between 45° and 50° in front and 50° and 55° behind (see Fig. 7).

The size of the foot is also important. A large horse with small, weak feet will not perform as well as the animal with a foot in proportion to his overall size.

The small foot with contracted heels interferes with the normal action of the 'frog'. At every step the pressure on the frog of a correctly trimmed hoof compresses the *plantar cushion*, aiding in the return of venous blood from the foot and lower part of the limb. Imbalance between the inner and outer heel of the foot causes an imbalance of stress on the joints of the limb, with all the ensuing problems caused by the uneven stress to weight-bearing surfaces.

Corns are another source of pain to the horse, though in many cases the pain can be termed sub-clinical – that is, there is no apparent lameness. Inspection of the wear of the shoe will often guide the intelligent owner to these problems, minor to begin with but, undetected, soon becoming major problems.

No farrier resents intelligent discussion and he will welcome helpful information as to the horse's way of going. The horse cannot talk, but you, the owner, by careful observation can often do it for him.

(a)   (b)

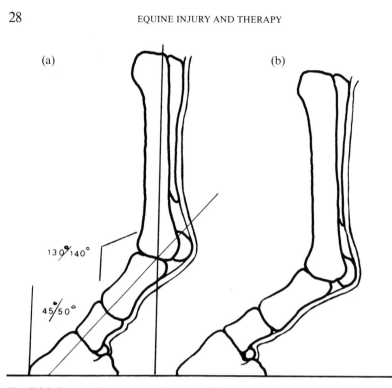

130°/140°

45°/50°

Fig. 7 (a) Correct foot to ground angles. (b) Incorrect foot to ground angle. Major cause: toe of foot left too long – the angle changes, with major injury to the suspensory apparatus of the limb.

Saddles

All too often, saddles do not fit; pads are then used to try to remedy the poor fit. Compression on the horse's spine causes pain, often resulting in his raising his head and going above the bit. The horse's reflex to avoid pain in the back is to hollow the back, which may cause severe bruising of the posterior spines of the vertebrae. Halftree saddles should be avoided at all costs; eventually, with wear, they distribute weight badly and can cause large, painful swellings in the centre of the back just below the end of the tree. These swellings may become infected, or the tissue may thicken as a protective mechanism, leaving an area of callus and scar tissue. Pressure on such an area always causes pain, and performance is badly impaired.

In 1891, Fred Smith, a veterinary surgeon sent to India to attend the horses of the Indian Cavalry, discovered most of the horses had sore backs; the reason was considered to be the poor performance of the men who rode the horses. Smith examined the saddle fit, and produced a design similar to the Cavalry Saddle of today. Within weeks of using these saddles with the weight well lateral to the spine, all sore backs had disappeared. (Smith's paper, entitled 'Manual of Saddles and Sore Backs', consists of 24 pages of logic.)

A wide gutter displaces the weight laterally, and allows the spine to function as a spring and absorb shock. Both rider weight and saddle weight should be evenly distributed – particularly in disciplines where the saddle is worn for long periods of time.

Like the stuffing in chairs and mattresses, saddle stuffing compresses eventually. Pads are no answer to an ill-fitting saddle, particularly pads that lie on and compress the area over the vertebral spines.

If you are in doubt about saddle fit, chalk the under-side – sit on the saddle, get off, remove the saddle, and look for pressure points. To measure the correct width, bend a piece of soft wire to the shape of your horse's back just behind the withers (old lead-covered electric cable is the most useful). Take this, with your saddle, to the saddler; he will do a much better job of re-stuffing.

Remember, without a comfortable back the horse cannot perform to his full potential. You make yourself comfortable. Your clothes fit. If they are uncomfortable, you can do something to make yourself comfortable: the horse cannot. Try carrying a heavy knapsack, unevenly loaded. You will be exhausted and cross before you have walked very far.

3 Examine to Help Your Vet

The aims of good treatment and rehabilitation are to determine the site of origin of the problem, to assist the normal repair process of the body by the use of the appropriate machine and to try to prevent recurrence by re-training and re-education.

The Veterinary Surgeons Act states quite clearly that no person other than a qualified veterinary surgeon or the owner of the animal may treat that animal unless so requested by the veterinary surgeon. To state this and then discuss an examination procedure would seem an anomaly, but every physiotherapist and owner should adopt a routine method of examination. Remember you are dealing with living tissue; the situation is not static; significant changes may have taken place since the vet's visit and it is necessary to observe and report on any findings or changes that may have taken place. This helps both the patient and the vet. Observation coupled with a good knowledge of the normal are of invaluable assistance when trying to solve a problem. The examiner must be able to visualize and appreciate shape, contours, range of movement, angle of limb parts. Always compare one side with the other – similar or dissimilar? Learn to appreciate through your fingers shape, texture, tension.

Soft tissue examination

The principles of soft tissue examination of the human can be adapted for animals. In the human, these are questions and observation; active movement; passive movement and resisted movement. You cannot question the animal, so you should question the person who looks after the animal. In the case of a horse, if one person rides and the other looks after the animal try to see both: each will help to paint a picture of the circumstances that gave rise to the condition needing treatment.

Type of questions that need to be asked even if you are the owner

(1) Was the horse fit enough for the competition, race or work demanded?

(2) Had there been any signs of stiffness or lack of willingness in performance prior to the accident/breakdown/incident?

(3) Any previous history of accident?

(4) Any noticeable heat in the effected leg over the past few months?

(5) Has the horse been reluctant to go downhill/to go uphill?

(6) Has the horse evaded the bit?

(7) Has the horse refused badly or consistently?

(8) Has the horse slipped on landing?

(9) Has the horse been cast recently?

(10) Has the horse travelled badly to a competition recently?

(11) Has the horse been kicked?

(12) Has the horse banged into a jump or been knocked by another horse while jumping?

(13) Has the horse felt resistant or one-sided when being schooled?

(14) Has the horse changed legs continuously while galloping?

(15) Has the horse shown signs of a cold back?

Observation

Do not have the horse moved. If rugged, do not have his rugs off; just look over the door of the box and note:

(1) Where is he standing in the box?

(2) Is his bed dug?

(3) Is he sitting on a wall? Are the walls marked, suggesting that he does sit against a wall?

(4) Has he rolled recently?

(5) What is his weight distribution: (a) even on all four legs; (b) resting one hind leg; (c) pointing a foreleg (note the angle of the pastern to the floor; is it similar in both forelegs/both hindlegs? – a difference in the angle may well mean uneven weight distribution).

When a head collar has been put on and the horse's quarters turned away from you, go to his head and make yourself known to him. Let him sniff you; rub his face or scratch his neck; let him get used to your smell and voice. Note the following:

(1) Condition of his coat: is it dull and lifeless, or shiny?

(2) Is his eye dull or bright?

(3) What is his general demeanour? Does he look as though he might be in pain?

Have the rugs removed. If the light is poor and if it is possible to do so, have the horse moved into a good light on an even floor. Deep straw, bad light and uneven floors cast shadows and change weight distribution, causing you to make mistakes. When he is moved into a good light, continue your observation.

Stand first on one side, then on the other, and look at the outline and muscle build; are both sides apparently similar? Stand directly in front of the head and look at the build of shoulders and forearms; wasting of the chest (pectoral) muscles is often missed. Stand behind and look at the quarters; is the top line even or uneven? Look at the development of the quarter muscles (gluteals), the position of the bony landmarks point of hip (tuber coxae) and jumpers bump (tuber sacrale) – use a milk crate if it is a tall horse. All these observations should be routine.

Even if you are only treating a forelimb, the accident which caused the damage to the forelimb may well have caused damage in some other area. Before starting the active part of your examination, feel the affected limb and note warmth, swelling and the texture of the structure under your fingers.

At this stage, unless you are treating a fracture, a complete breakdown of tendon, post-operative repair or some condition that requires minimal movement, you are ready to start the active part of the examination. The animal should be walked away and back, trotted away and back. You should position yourself so that it is possible to see movement from in front, behind and the side. Lameness denotes pain or limb disfunction; learn to listen for an irregular beat denoting lameness, as well as being able to see lameness.

Active movement

Active movement involves muscle, joint and ligament. From the pattern of the walk and trot, you should be able to decide not necessarily the structure at fault, but at least in which area of the body pain is being experienced – left side, right side, forequarter, hindquarter, spine.

Some typical movement patterns

A lame horse usually nods his head as he trots. If lame in front, his head usually drops as the sound leg meets the ground, the head rising, sometimes sharply, as the painful leg meets the ground. Lameness arising from the shoulders or withers can cause a rather pottery short stride in front, almost as if the horse is tied in at the elbow. Hind-leg lameness may cause a horse to lower his head as the painful leg meets the ground, while discomfort in the loins (*thoraco lumbar*) area produces a shuffly hind-leg action with the hind feet tracking only half the normal distance forward. In some cases this is more apparent on one side than the other. In many cases the toes of the hind feet are dragged along the ground, almost as though the hock is not functioning correctly.

The back

If you have any suspicion that the horse is suffering from pain arising from his back, after the active phase return the horse to the stable or an enclosed area and proceed to look at the back movements. Movements in a horse's back are not very great, but a horse with a normal spine is capable of *dorsiflexion* (hollowing), *ventroflexion* (arching) and *side-flexion* (Fig. 8).

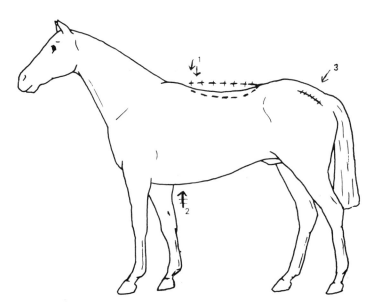

Fig. 8 Normal movements in the back of the average horse: (1) pressure behind the withers on both sides causes *dipping* or *dorsiflexion*; (2) pressure behind the girth causes *humping* or *ventroflexion*; (3) drawing the finger firmly down the quarters as on the diagram causes *side-flexion*. Worry when one or more movement is absent or causes obvious pain.

Dorsiflexion: stimulate by pressing down on either side of the back just behind the withers. The horse will normally dip his back.

Ventroflexion: stimulate by putting your hand underneath the abdomen and pressing just behind the girth line. The horse will normally arch his back.

Side-flexion: stimulate by running your fingers along either side of the spine, first on one side and then on the other, approximately a hand span from the spine. The horse will normally bend away from the pressure.

Neck: turn the head and see if the horse can reach his rib cage with his nose. Reluctance to turn the neck (*cervical spine*) or an inability denotes a problem.

Most horses, like most humans, are one sided, but it is very easy to ascertain a lack of movement or reluctance to perform movement. Your examination should take place before the horse has been exercised. After exercise, due to the increased circulatory flow, stiffness may wear off, the pain diminish and your diagnostic picture become far from clear.

Passive movement

This is the approved method of investigating joints other than the *vertebral column* and the supporting ligaments of the joints. By manually performing the normal joint movement, you eliminate muscle involvement. By stressing the end of movement range, you put strain on the joint capsule and associated ligaments. Pain illicited on passive examination must logically arise from the joint being stressed; it then remains to determine which ligament or ligaments are involved. To employ this part of the examination correctly, a very precise knowledge of the movement of each joint is necessary, as is the ability to stress one joint at a time. A classic example of passive testing is the hock flexion test for spavin.

When you have tested all the joints in the quarter of the body in which you consider the injury lies, note the pastern angle of the legs. If you consider that the weight distribution is uneven, ask an assistant to pick up the opposite leg and note the angle of the pastern of the leg on which the horse is now forced to put weight. Is it similar to that which the opposite leg adopted? In the fore limb, if the angle changes and the fetlock drops, there could be a problem with either the *superficial* and/or *deep digital flexor tendon* and/or the *suspensory ligament* (see Fig. 11).

In the human, we pass from active and passive movement to resisted movement.

Resisted movement

Resisted movement is performed in such a way that no joint action takes place, the resistance being applied to produce *isometric contraction* (isometric = contraction of muscles without movement) of individual muscles. If pain is illicited, the damage (lesion) is considered to lie within the contracting muscle. The only method of invoking isometric contraction in the horse is by the use of a muscle stimulator. First advocated by Sir Charles Strong, this method will often assist in isolating the muscle involved. Such an examination takes time, and this is where a physiotherapist can be of great help to a veterinary surgeon.

Once the site of the origin of the pain and the type of tissue involved are established and the secondary damage noted, treatment can begin. If you are a physiotherapist, discuss with the vet in charge the treatment programme, giving your reasons. If the vet agrees, explain the regime to the owner. Discuss bitting, dentistry, saddle fitting, shoeing; all are part of rehabilitation.

Remember, the aims of treatment are to determine the site of the origin of the problem, to assist the normal repair process of the body by the use of the appropriate machine, and to try to prevent recurrence by retraining and re-education.

X-ray and scanning as aids to diagnosis

The pictures supplied by X-rays are dependent on the density of the objects in their path; therefore, unless specialist dyes are injected the only picture the X-ray apparatus provides clearly is of bone. Diagnostically, it is invaluable for bone-associated conditions, arthritis, fractures, the state of bone growth, decrease in bone density, bone tumours, and so on.

Severe back pain in the human caused by ruptured discs or problems within the spinal canal will not show on plain X-ray and these conditions are diagnosed by injecting dye, or more recently a specialist type of oil, into the spinal canal and then taking X-ray pictures. The dye outlines the structures and it is relatively easy to establish the level and extent of pressure causing the problem. This type of X-ray is called a *reticulogram* or *mylogram*.

Recent advances in machine design have produced the scanner. At present, the ultrasound scanner is used primarily, within the equine field, to diagnose pregnancy in the brood mare. An exciting new breakthrough is the ability to scan the structures of the limbs. In the foreseeable future, it will be possible to determine the extent of damage in the deep and superficial flexor tendons and the suspensory ligament.

The technique is non-invasive; there are no radiation problems as there are with X-ray. From the therapy point of view it should, using scanners, be possible to evaluate the repair within a structure and to establish the best possible treatment protocol. Scanning is rapidly replacing mylography in the human field.

Isotope scanning

To X-ray the spine of the horse requires general anasthesia – by injecting a radioactive isotope into the circulatory system, then scanning the animal with a gamma camera, it is possible to locate the 'hot spots', or areas of unusual activity, in the skeleton and so diagnose fracture sites and other problems.

NMR scanning

NMR scanning – Nuclear Magnetic Resonance scanning – is the latest achievement in the medical diagnostic field, the apparatus allowing a three-dimensional picture of the scanned area to be achieved.

Within the foreseeable future, all these pieces of apparatus will be available at veterinary research centres.

Heart rate computers

The usefulness of the ability to monitor the heart rate during exercise and recovery is well established and understood in the human athlete. In the horse, the significance of the readings logged and their use in interval and associated methods of training is the subject of considerable controversy.

Heart rate increases not only during exercise (it will be suggested that heart rates be monitored during therapeutic swimming sessions) but also as a result of pain.

As already stated, effective treatment is not possible without accurate knowledge of the site of injury. The ability to examine an animal described as having 'lost form', but having no heat or other obvious clinical signs or findings, and to determine, by the use of a heart rate monitor, the changes in heart rate during palpitation, passive joint movement and muscle testing, can only be of benefit.

There is a large variation of heartbeats to the minute within the acceptable normal range. It is useful to know the heart rate of individual animals, before loss of form or suspected injury.

Many large training yards log individual temperatures daily; unfortunately, as yet few bother with heart rates – even if the normal resting heart rate is not on record and is slightly elevated due to pain, there will still be a significant temporary rise when pain is increased during examination.

Expected equine heart rate readings compiled by the manufacturers of the EQB meter.

		Rates per minute
Standing		40
Walking		80
Trotting	(234 metres/minute)	120
Trotting	(290 metres/minute)	140
Galloping	(348 metres/minute)	160
Galloping	(500 metres/minute)	200

Heart beats have been recorded as high as 285 beats per minute (bpm). Rates of 250 bpm are not uncommon in racing Thoroughbreds. Old horses (15 years and up) have much higher rates during exercise; young horses in training for the first time also have much higher working heart rates.

Remember, *changes* in your horse's heart rate day-to-day and week-to-week are as important as the absolute rate at any time; therefore, you must keep records. Every horse is an individual and will not have the same exact response as another to exercise.

Horses' heart rates can and do change very suddenly, especially from 30 to 130 beats per minute. Such changes do not indicate a problem with your heart rate computer.

These figures were obtained from trainers using the EQB and from the results of Frederick Fregin, formerly a professor in equine cardiology at Cornell Veterinary School and now at the University of Pennsylvania New Bolton Center.

Note: heart rates do not relate to work or fitness alone; they are affected by fear, excitement, and pain. A sick horse (for example, a horse with a temperature) will have higher than normal heart rates. Also, if the heart rates of your horse do not coincide with the above, see the trouble-shooting guide in your Equistat-user instruction manual, and *check your horse!* Check the tack, the legs and feet and shoes, etc.

Below are some comments on expected equine heart rate readings for horses aged 3 to 14 years, as supplied by EQB (rates for horses younger or older than that are generally higher).

Standing: resting rates in the stall can range anywhere from as low as 25 bpm, to 120 bpm if the horse is startled by a strange person or object in the stable. When tacked up, with a rider, most horses range from 40 to 60 bpm (or higher if the horse is anticipating work).

Jogging: a horse that has been ridden for at least six months will usually jog slowly (trotting 234 metres/minute) between 115 bpm to 130bpm. The same horse may do an open trot (290 metres/minute) with a heart rate as high as 155, averaging around 140 bpm. Gentle inclines seem to add about 10 to 15 bpm to these averages and steep inclines as much as 50 bpm, usually around 35 bpm.

Cantering: an *easy* hand canter (320 metres/minute) will often exhibit in some horses a *lower* heart rate than an open jog, the range, once again in a reasonably fit individual, being 130 to 155 bpm.

Galloping: in hand, but not too quickly (under a two minute lick), 348 metres/minute, a reasonably fit horse will average around 165 bpm, often on a flat uniform surface as low as 150 or, depending upon attitude, as high as 180 or 190.

Very fast working or galloping: 500 metres/minute or a two minute lick or faster. Depending upon the horse's stage of conditioning, ability, attitude, lameness, and other general health, after going on the initial 1/8th mile (in which hearts will peak sometimes 30 to 40 bpm above what they will then even out to), 200 beats per minute is a good average. Very fit, talented horses often will work 3/8th mile in 36 seconds with a maximum rate under 200 bpm and recover to 100 bpm in a minute or less. Longer works will cause higher maximum rates and longer recovery times.

Note: heart rates in excess of 250 beats per minute indicate some kind of exercise intolerance, whether because of attitude, health, age, condition, lameness, tack, or other problems.

4 Common Sites of Injury in the Horse

Commonsense first aid is the priority at the time of accident. Then, draw breath. There is an unfortunate tendency to rush in with every aid available in a frantic endeavour to achieve immediate recovery. Unfortunately, this approach often exacerbates the problem, one 'aid' reversing the effects of another and the over-treating of an area never giving the natural healing processes a chance. Brilliant blistering of areas has been achieved by treatment overdoses! Try to take an unemotional, rational view; get a diagnosis, calculate the approximate time required for recovery, choose the best apparatus available, and go to work. If repair is achieved in a time shorter than expected, it is a bonus.

Listed in the table below are the most common sites of injury in the horse (see Fig. 9), the aims of treatment, the machines to achieve the aims in order of *professional preference*, and the names of the muscles that may require stimulation after the injury described. For accuracy of muscle stimulation, refer to Figs 19–28.

Note: all machines have an analgesic, pain-killing effect. The absence of pain is not an indication of complete recovery.

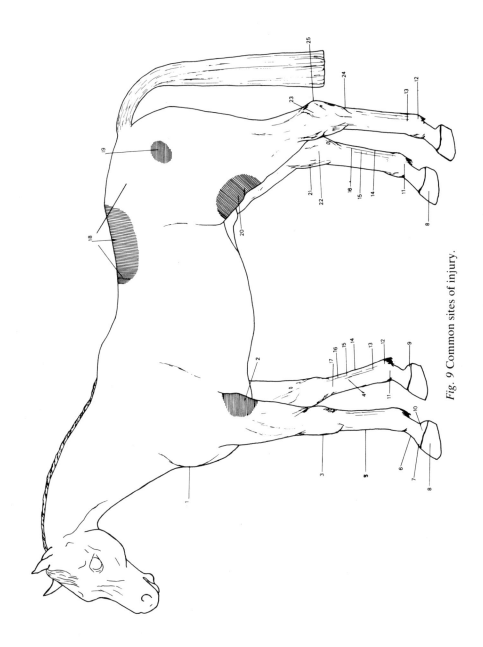

Fig. 9 Common sites of injury.

Condition	Aims of treatment after first aid	Suggested machines	Muscles probably involved. Stimulate
1. *Bicepital bursitis* Inflammation of the bursa lying in the bicepital groove near the point of the shoulder. As the foreleg retracts the bursa is compressed, with resultant pain and shortening of stride. Not usually a 'nodding' lameness	Reduce inflammation Reduce pain	Ultrasound (3 MHz head) Magnetic field therapy Electrovet/Ionicare Massage	Deltoid Triceps Pectorals
2. *Elbow* Capsulitis of the joint following overstretching injury. Bruising (capped elbow) may be due to insufficient bedding or the horse catching and bruising his elbow at exercise.	Establish and remove cause Reduce inflammation Reduce swelling Maintain full range of movement	Ultrasound (3 MHz head) Magnetic field therapy Electrovet/Ionicare Passive stretching	Extensor Carpi radialis Superficial pectoral
3. *Knee* (a) Direct trauma with bruising and/or lacerations.	(a) Reduce swelling Avoid infection Avoid proud flesh Maintain full mobility	Cold between treatments, e.g. Bonner-type bandage Laser and compression Ultrasound Passive flexion with fetlock flexed	Deltoid Pectorals Triceps

Condition	Aims of treatment after first aid	Suggested machines	Muscles probably involved. Stimulate
(b) Capsulitis due to excessive stress.	(b) Reduce inflammation Maintain full movement	Ultrasound followed by Electrovet/Ionicare Magnetic field therapy	
(c) Flake fractures may occur as the result of hyper-extension (loose bodies).	(c) After surgical removal of chips Promote healing Avoid adhesions	Laser Passive movements with fetlock flexed	
N.B. X-ray knee problems.		ULTRASOUND MAY BE CONTRA-INDICATED	
4. *Splint bone* (a) Inflammation of the interossious ligament between the splint and cannon bone. Fusion of the two bones is the end result. Causes: concussion, trauma, uneven shoeing with resultant uneven stress.	To promote early fusion with minimal bone formation Maintain fitness	Cold between treatments, e.g. Bonner-type bandage Laser Magnetic field therapy Electrovet/Ionicare Massage ULTRASOUND MAY BE CONTRA-INDICATED Swim	
(b) Fracture of bone, usually by direct trauma, may require surgical removal.			
5. *Sore shins* (Fig. 10) (a) Inflammation of the periosteum on the	Reduce inflammation Promote healing	Cold between treatments, e.g. Bonner-type	

(b) Hairline fractures through the front of the cannon bone. Causes include concussion, direct trauma, nutritional bone diseases. NB. Sore shins are more common in the fore than the hindlimbs. Severe cases may 'buck'. X-ray is advisable to determine severity.	Maintain fitness Reduce concussion	Laser Magnetic field therapy Electrovet/Ionicare Massage ULTRASOUND MAY BE CONTRA-INDICATED Swim Specialist pads, e. g. E–Z Strider/Sorbothane
6. *High ringbone* Unwanted bone is laid down at the upper end of the short pastern.	Reduce inflammation Minimise new bone growth Reduce concussion	The value of machine therapy is debatable Try Ultrasound or magnetic field therapy Swim Specialist pads, e. g. E–Z Strider/Sorbothane
7. *Low ringbone* Unwanted bone is laid down at the lower end of the short pastern. Unless the new bone interferes with joint movement, it is of no consequence.		
8. *Sandcrack* A split in the outer wall of the hoof may involve the coronary band. Caused by direct trauma, badly trimmed unshod feet, injury to the coronary band.	Promote healthy hoof growth Specialist shoeing to support crack	Laser to coronary band
9. *Overreach* A cut or cuts caused by striking the heel of the forefoot with the toe of the hindfoot.	Prevent infection Promote healing	Laser Ultrasound (3 MHz head) Magnetic field therapy

Condition	Aims of treatment after first aid	Suggested machines	Muscles probably involved. Stimulate
10. *Sidebones* Unwanted bone formation in the lateral cartilages, possibly as a result of concussion. If the bone growth interferes with the movement between the foot and short pastern, specialist shoeing is called for.	Promote healing with minimal bone formation	Ultrasound (3 MHz head) Magnetic field therapy	
11. *Fetlock joint* (a) Capsulitis due to sprain	(a) Reduce inflammation Maintain full movement	Cold between treatments, e.g. Bonner-type bandage Ultrasound (3 MHz head) Electrovet/Ionicare Magnetic field therapy Massage Passive stretching Swim	Deltoid Triceps Pectorals
(b) Bruising due to direct trauma.	(b) Reduce bruising.		
(c) Degenerative arthritis can occur in older horses.	(c) Improve the integrity of the joint capsules	Ultrasound (3 MHz head) Magnetic field therapy Passive stretching Swim	
(d) Fractures of the pastern or lower end of the cannon will involve the joint	(d) Promote healing	Magnetic field therapy	

12. **Sesamoid bones** (a) Inflammation of one or both of the proximal sesamoids. Often concurrent with problems in the fetlock joint.	(a) Reduce inflammation Maintain full movement Maintain fitness in acute stage	Cold between treatments, e.g. Bonner-type bandage Laser Ultrasound Magnetic field therapy Electrovet/Ionicare Massage Passive stretching Swim
(b) Fracture of one or both of the proximal sesamoids. X-ray is advisable.	(b) Promote healing	Magnetic field therapy
13. **Windgalls (windpuffs)** There is a distension of the synovial sheath between either the suspensory ligament and cannon bone or the long pastern and ligament joining the sesamoids. Cause: overstress of the limb, concussion or incorrect angulation of joint of the foot and pastern. NB. Tends to be more common in the hind than forelegs.	Reduce inflammation before the condition becomes chronic Remove cause if possible	Ultrasound Magnetic field therapy Elastic stocking when stood in

Condition	Aims of treatment after first aid	Suggested machines	Muscles probably involved. Stimulate
14, 15. *Flexor tendons and/or suspensory ligament* (Figs 11 and 12) The superficial, the deep, or both may be involved. Partial or complete rupture may occur. Bowing is present (Fig. 12). In all cases, support of the fetlock joint is reduced. Severe case may be supported by casting.	Support the area Reduce swelling Reduce inflammation Promote healing Maintain muscle strength in shoulder	Support and cold, e.g. Bonner-type bandage; follow with tube-grip Ultrasound (3 MHz head) Electrovet/Ionicare Massage Laser with Electrovet/ Ionicare and massage Magnetic field therapy with Electrovet/Ionicare and massage Magnetic field therapy will penetrate a cast – no other machine will be of use if a cast is used	Deltoid Triceps Pectorals Supraspinatus Infraspinatus Extensor carpi ulnaris
16. *Check ligament* Damage can occur in association with tendon and/or suspensory injuries, or as a separate issue.	Reduce inflammation Promote healing Maintain fitness	Treat as for tendons	Stimulate as for tendons
17. *Speedy cut* Cuts caused by striking one leg with shoe or hoof of another leg.	Prevent infection Promote healing	Laser Ultrasound (3 MHz head) Magnetic field therapy	

18. *Thoraco lumbar and/or pelvic problems* Opinions vary widely as to the reasons for damage in the spine and pelvis. The problems are thought to be ligament tears, with associated muscle weakness. Fractures (hairline cracks in particular) have been observed in many bone specimens, along with arthritic and other body changes.	Reduce pain Re-educate muscles Re-educate movement	Ultrasound (1 MHz head) Magnetic field therapy Deep massage Swim	Longissimus Glutei
19. *Trochenteric bursitis* The bursa lies under the tendon of the middle gluteal muscle and above the greater trochanter of the femur. Pressure caused by the contraction of the gluteals compresses the bursa, giving rise to shortening of stride and, on occasions, severe lameness.	Reduce inflammation Maintain muscle strength Re-educate movement after reduction of pain	Ultrasound (1 MHz head) Magnetic field therapy Deep massage Muscle stimulation after reduction of pain	Gluteal muscles Semimembranous Semitendinosus Biceps femoris
20. *Stifle joint* The stifle joint corresponds to the human knee; the patella corresponds to the human knee cap. Most stifle problems result from the patella deviating from its normal anatomical position. These movements may cause the joint to 'lock'. Any dislocation of the patella causes extensive ligament stretching and associated muscle weakness.	Reduce dislocation if present Reduce inflammation if present Maintain muscle strength	Ultrasound (3 MHz head) Laser Massage Muscle stimulation	Semitendinosus Semimembranous Biceps femoris Vastus lateralis

Condition	Aims of treatment after first aid	Suggested machines	Muscles probably involved. Stimulate
21, 22. *Spavin* Bog spavin – capsulitis of the hock. The result of stress or poor conformation. Bone spavin – unwanted bone forms, usually on the inner surface of the hock, interfering with articulation of the joint; or there is erosion of the articular surfaces followed by new bone growth. N.B. In the author's experience, the hock is the most unpredictable joint to treat. Treat all cases, whatever the condition, with great caution.	Reduce inflammation Reduce inflammation Maintain joint range	Laser Electrovet/Ionicare Massage	
23. *Thoroughpin* A swelling of the sheath of the deep flexor tendon of the hock due to trauma or strain.	Reduce swelling	Cold (Bonner-type bandage) Electrovet/Ionicare Ultrasound (3 MHz head), with caution Massage	
24. *Curb* Thickening of the plantar tarsal ligament, usually caused by over-exertion. Poor conformation is a contributory factor.	Reduce inflammation Control swelling	Cold (Bonner-type bandage) Laser Ultrasound (3 MHz head) Electrovet/Ionicare Massage Swim	

25. *Capped hock* Swelling of the bursa over the point of the hock, usually caused by trauma or sitting against the box wall.	Reduce inflammation	Cold (Bonner-type bandage) Ultrasound Electrovet/Ionicare	
Bruised or torn muscles If left untreated, bruising in a muscle will 'scar'; that is, a dense area of fibrous tissue with no elastic properties will form. This will reduce the efficiency of surrounding muscle tissue and, when the muscle is at full stretch, the tissue above or below the scar will be over-stressed and in its turn will tear.	Reduce the bruise (haematoma) Maintain maximal muscle efficiency Prevent adhesions	Cold Laser Ultrasound Magnetic field therapy Electrovet/Ionicare Massage	Stimulate muscle groups

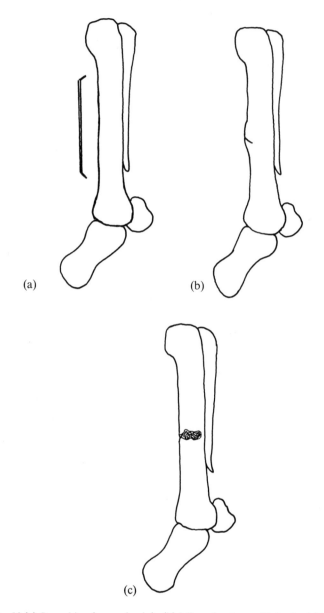

Fig. 10 (a) Sore shins (area of pain). (b) Micro-fracture with buck. (c) Stress fracture.

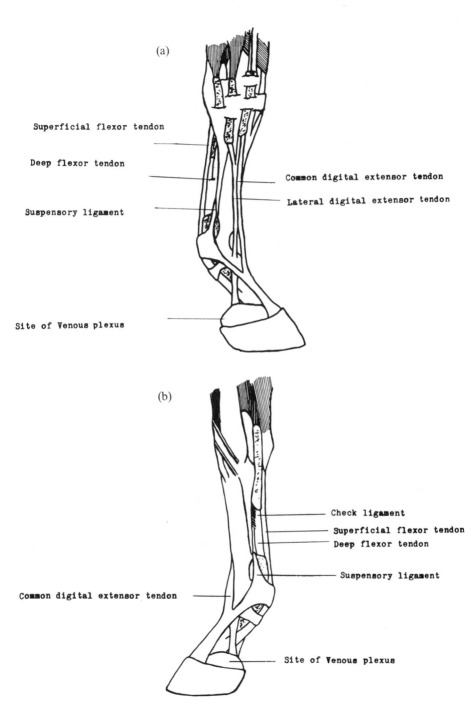

Fig. 11 Diagram of the tendons of the foreleg: (a) medial aspect, and (b) lateral aspect.

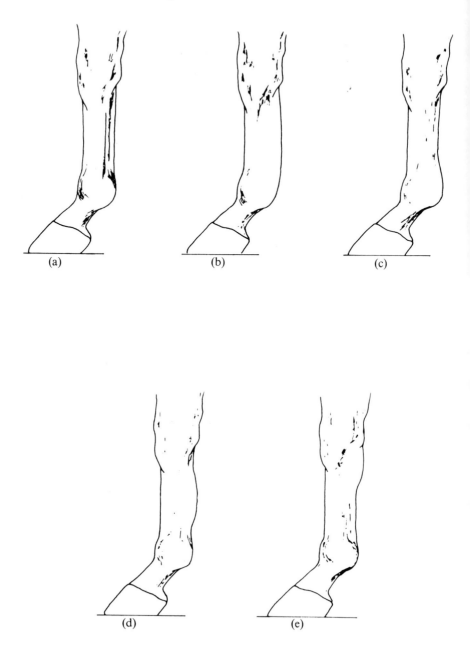

Fig. 12 Tendon injuries: (a) normal tendon contour, (b) bowed tendon, (c) low bow, (d) middle bow, and (e) high bow.

5 The Machines and Their Uses

Treatment can only be effective after accurate diagnosis.

Examination and subsequent diagnosis require the skills of the veterinary profession, with their ability not only to question, look, feel and smell, but also nerve block X-ray, blood test, scan and scope – the latter both for the respiratory system and certain joints. All these aids are within the field of general practice. Obviously serious problems require the added facilities of the veterinary research establishments.

Haphazard treatment without a diagnosis can be costly in both time and money, and in many cases is ineffective.

Contrary to general belief, it is rare to find a member of the veterinary profession who will not co-operate with responsible, knowledgeable machine-owners. Quite reasonably, it is annoying for the professional to be called in to sort out problems caused by irresponsible treatments.

Unfortunately, there are no set 'treatment recipes' for musculoskeletal conditions, as there are for 'drug therapy'. Relate to yourself: if you have bronchitis, the doctor gives you a perscription for an antibiotic, and provided you, as the patient, stick to the dosage, you will be well within a calculated time. Sprain an ankle, and there is no set time; recovery depends on the degree of the injury, the ability to receive the correct treatment at the correct time, and your ability to re-educate the movement pattern lost as a result of the pain. Remember, pain inhibits movement. The effects of the pain are best described by the vicious circle of injury.

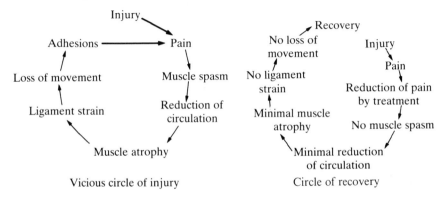

Vicious circle of injury   Circle of recovery

All that can be suggested are the aims of treatment. It is up to
individuals to choose the machines required, or to make the best use of
the machines they already have.

First aid

Compress the area. Support the area. Keep the patient warm.

In principle, all injuries should be seen by a vet (horse) or doctor
(human). In the event of there being no professional help on hand, the
owner/trainer must take the responsibility and do the best that he/she
can in the circumstances.

A *first aid box* is a must. The box should be kept stocked and always
stored in the same place. All too often, the famous 'someone' has
moved the kit, and that 'someone' is always missing in a crisis; or the
box has been raided, and the necessary items are missing.

The minimum contents should comprise:

Cotton wool
Suitable disinfectant
Bandages – stretch, crepe, elastic and triangular
Lint
Gamgee
Elastoplast (or Band Aid in USA)
A roll of elastic bandage and a box of elastoplast dressings
Scissors
Melolin dressing
Jelonet dressing
Animalintex

Useful additions are:

Wound dressing powder
Cold bandages
Purple spray
Iodine (old fashioned!)
Micropore tape
Arnica ointment
Pack of sterile saline solution
50 cc syringe in a sterile pack with suitable needles to withdraw the
saline
Cold bandages in packs

Animalintex is carried by most people. It has a place, but for
immediate first aid melolin dressings may be as good if not better.

Clean. Always clean to reduce the risk of infection in an open wound. It is essential to clean the wound thoroughly, however difficult this may be at the time of injury. The removal of all foreign bodies, mud, hair, grit, pays dividends, the risk of secondary infection being reduced to a minimum. The principle of cleaning and sterilising wounds was enforced by Florence Nightingale at the time of the Crimean War; human medicine took a great step forward!

Cover. Open wounds need a dressing – preferably the type that, when removed, will not stick. For this, Melolin is ideal.

Compress. Compression equals even pressure over and around the injured area, and is aimed at reducing haemorrhage – that is, the loss of blood and fluid from the injured tissues. Cotton wool or a gamgee pad should be placed over the dressing, and an appropriate bandage applied. Bandaging has two functions:

(1) To hold the dressing in place.
(2) Support.

The injured tissue is unable to fulfil normal functions; the bandage can assist by taking strain off adjacent tissues temporarily having to take over the activity of the injured area. Bandaging is an art in itself.

It should be noted that almost as much damage can be done by bad bandaging as by no bandaging at all (see Appendix I).

Cold. Cold assists in reducing the risk of continued bleeding (*haemorrhage*) by causing a temporary constriction of the blood vessels. Movement should be restricted to a minimum for 24 hours after injury.

Treatment

Following diagnosis, with the knowledge of the extent and nature of the problem, a programme of treatment and management can be initiated.

Early re-establishment of an adequate circulatory flow is essential for healing. Should the circulation be drastically reduced, tissue death (*ischaemia*) may occur. It is for this reason bandages must be checked every few hours in the immediate post injury period.

The human reports pre-ischaemic pain, and observation shows 'blue' fingers or toes. The horse has no method, other than removing his bandages with his teeth, to show discomfort. All too often, bandages are covered with Cribbox to discourage removal. A horse that is comfortable usually leaves his bandages alone.

Massage

One of the oldest and most effective treatments is that of massage. Described as the use of the hands and fingers to affect the soft tissues, it is an art; and, like a good groom, good masseurs with sensitive fingers are worth their weight in gold. The ability to detect differing tensions in tissues through the fingers is a valuable diagnostic aid. Correctly given, massage influences the venous return and thereby provides for a more rapid removal of waste products, whether they have been produced by injury or by exercise. Grooming is a type of massage that, done correctly, particularly with a body brush or wisp, stimulates the circulation.

Massage before exercise is of great benefit. For example, athletes rub (massage) their limbs before they begin the active part of their warm-up.

After exercise, horses used to be wisped dry – that is, massaged dry; today, they are often just washed off. The benefits of this compared with a good wisping must be questionable. Try a cold bath yourself after a long cross-country run; stand still for twelve hours, and see how you feel.

Massage is more easily performed if a lubricant is used. There is then very little pull on the hair of the coat or the skin, and no possibility of causing pain.

Hand massage

There are several types of massage strokes which can be applied.

Efflurage

The hands are moulded around or over the tissues, and a firm pressure is applied as the hands are pushed away from the operator's body, the direction of the stroke being as directly parallel to the return of venous blood as is possible. At the end of the stroke, the hands are drawn back towards the operator with less pressure, and the next stroke is effected.

Uses: reduction of swelling (*oedema*) after other massage strokes; after strenuous exercise.

Kneading

The hands are placed over the bulk of the muscle; the tissues are pressed inward and then lifted away from the underlying structures, cupped in the palm of the hand.

Uses: dispersal of a haematoma; breakdown of adhesions in the muscle post injury; reducing muscle tension after exertion. Follow with *efflurage*.

Friction

Friction is a localised massage; the forefinger reinforced by the second finger of one hand is placed over the area requiring treatment. The movement is small and should be performed in such a way that the stroke sweeps across the linear direction of the underlying fibres. The finger should not slip over the top of the skin when frictioning; if this occurs, a blister will result. The skin and underlying tissues must literally be moved one over the other.

Uses: breakdown of scar tissue, breakdown of adhesions; for tendon injuries. Follow with *efflurage*.

Mechanical massagers

Mechanical massagers are now available both as hand-held units (Plate 2) and specialised pads. The latter can be adapted to fit almost any area of the horse (or human).

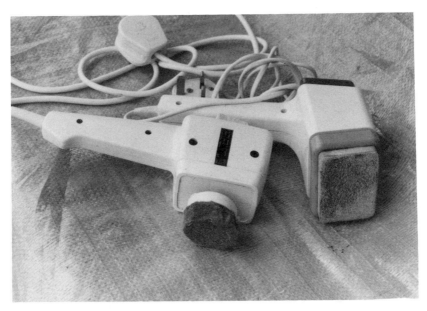

Plate 2 Hand-held mechanical massagers.

The effect of these machines is one of vibration. Patients tolerate the sensation well, and the machines are of great benefit if used sensibly. Electrically driven, either from the mains or from a portable battery mounted on a trolley, they have a variable depth of vibration. It is suggested that an animal be allowed to become accustomed to the noise before the machine is used.

Hold the pad in position, rather than strap and leave, when first starting to use, in order to allow the animal to become accustomed to the sensation. This should be minimal at first. The vibration strength can then be varied according to the individual case. It is recommended that the machines be used for approximately 30 minutes at each session. The cheapest is the Pifco, hand-held vibrator. Best results are obtained in limbs of the horse if a tube-grip stocking is applied and the machines moved on top of the stocking.

Uses: pre and post strenuous exercise or competition work; all cases of soft tissue injury; adherent scarring; filled joints, bruises; windgalls; etc.

All types of massage are passive techniques, and massage cannot be considered a substitute for muscular contraction. It is usually used in conjunction with other forms of treatment. The latest innovation is underwater massage in the form of a *jacuzzi* – a tub of warm water containing jets which are played against the submerged tissues. A leg tub is available for horses.

Kits can be purchased to fit into normal bath tubs for the human sufferer.

Cold/ice/water

Cold can be used as first aid and as a treatment. Utilised for first aid, due to *vaso-constriction*, *haematoma* formation is controlled, *oedema* reduced and there is a mild analgesic effect. First aid can be applied in a number of ways.

Commercially produced sachets. These contain non-toxic gels; after refrigeration they remain flexible yet cold for up to three hours. Some have carrying cases which ensure they remain cold for five hours after removal from the refrigerator, enabling them to be part of a mobile first aid kit when travelling.

Commercially produced bandages. These bandages, impregnated with gel, cool rapidly down to 34°F when exposed to air and remain cool for up to three hours. They are re-usable (Plate 3).

Bonner bandages. The great advantage of Bonner bandages is their twofold effect: support and cold. The fabric has stretch characteristics and remains cold after refrigeration for 15 minutes.

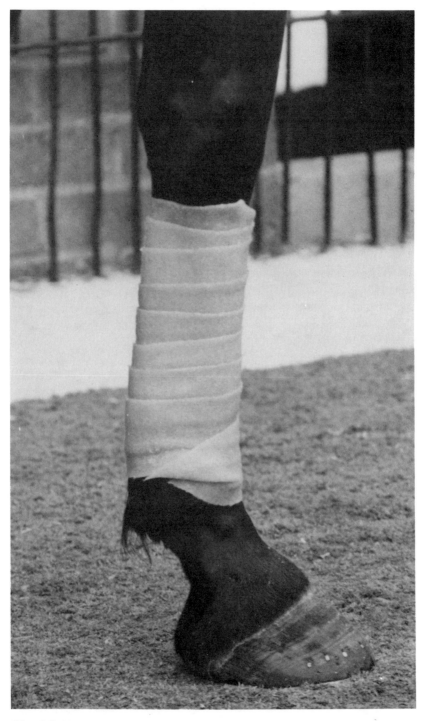

Plate 3 Cold bandage.

The ice crystals melt slowly after the bandage is applied. Skin temperature under the bandage reaches the therapeutic range of 6°C. As well as home use, the bandage provides instant cold for first aid when packed in a thermal bag and taken to outside events (Plate 4).

Frozen gamgee or cotton wool. Gamgee or a thick pad of cotton wool can be soaked in water, shaped to the injured area, frozen in a deep freeze, and then bandaged into place. Several made up at one time ensure a constant supply, and the necessity to replace also ensures that the injury is checked at regular intervals. Towels soaked in ice cold water, wrung out and then bandaged into place are also useful.

Precautions

Do not place frozen substances in direct contact with the skin, as this may cause ice burn. Do not leave ice in situ for more than a maximum of 30 minutes, or the tissues may freeze to death. This is the advantange of using iced gamgee, cotton wool or towels: they melt reasonably rapidly. If it is considered that there is a major nerve involvement, *do not use cold*: the tissues might reach an unacceptable level of chill, and die.

Cold as therapy

For years, hosing has been advocated for leg injuries. Horses have stood in streams or walked in the sea. All have a cooling effect; the two latter also have a compression effect due to the pressure of the water. The response is more subtle if ice is employed.

The physiological effects of ice therapy

Research has shown the following tissue response:

(1) *Vaso-constriction*, followed by
(2) Deep tissue *vaso-dilatation*.
(3) Reduction in *muscle spasm*.
(4) A limited *thermal analgesic*.

Of these, the first two are important in the treatment of the horse.

Vaso-constriction

During the first 4–6 minutes of cold application, the area undergoes a

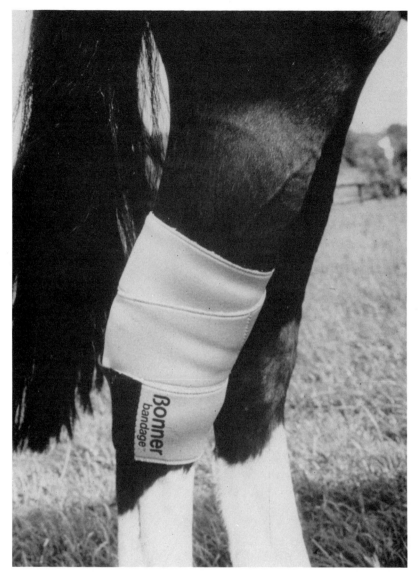

Plate 4 Cold bandage.

reduction of blood flow. The inflammatory reaction in the area is temporarily curtailed.

Vaso-dilatation

If the cold application continues for longer than 6–10 minutes, there is a deep tissue vaso-dilatation lasting from 6–12 minutes. Known as 'hunter's rush', this response is a thermo-regulatory response to the unacceptable cold, or thermal insult, to the area. Vaso-constriction then recurs, followed by a vaso-dilatation in a 15–30 minute cycle. By this method, an increased circulatory flow through the area is established. Hosing does not have the same effect, although it undoubtedly causes local vaso-constriction.

Methods of employing ice/water therapy

The limb can be immersed in a container, which is then filled with water to which crushed ice is added. A plastic bucket or dustbin will serve, but the purpose-built aqua boots, or 'horse wellies' as they are affectionately known, are the most practical method of application. The aqua boot has the added advantage of an attached compressor mechanism; the water in the boot can be agitated producing underwater massage. In some yards, this type of underwater massage has been effected by using a vacuum cleaner hose with the vacuum cleaner mechanism reversed! The Boot is the more practical. Sea salts, epsom salts or other additives are sometimes used in place of ice, but there is no proof that their addition is beneficial.

Ice massage

For areas where submersion is impractical, ice massage can be employed. Ice cubes are messy, hard to hold and numb the fingers. The most useful method is to freeze a paper cup of water with a lolly stick in the centre. Holding the stick, you can utilize the frozen end without freezing off your own fingers – useful for working over bruised areas on the trunk.

Treatment times

Hosing, aqua boots: up to 20 minutes, two or three times a day. Iced water: 15 minutes, two or three times a day. When using ice, make certain the horse is warm himself.

After an application in water, towel dry (working up the limb). A hair dryer is a great help, particularly if bandages are to be re-applied and are not of the glentona type.

Uses: these methods can be safely used for all soft tissue injuries – that is, sprains, strains, tears, filled joints.

Note: iced water in aqua boots is used as a routine by some owners for their competition horses. It is particularly popular with those who own trotters and with some of the show jumpers. The effects can easily be obtained by using a hand massage unit, but it may be that there is warmth in the legs of these types of competition animals due to some deeper structural problem. The immersion in water will reduce the warmth, thus allowing their owners to be fooled into thinking that there is no problem. The cold will also have a mild analgesic effect, and therefore any sign of discomfort or lameness could well be supressed.

Heat

Heat can be applied either to the surface of the body by specialist lamps (superficial heat), or by employing a high frequency alternating current which heats the deeper structures (deep heat).

Superficial heat

Infra red lamps are a source of radiant energy. This energy penetrates the skin (epidermis) into the underlying tissue (dermis), and is experienced as warmth.

Effects of superficial heat on the tissues.

There is a rise in temperature throughout the area at which the heat is directed. This temperature rise increases the circulation. As the warmth becomes unacceptably high, the local blood vessels dilate in order to try to lose heat, with a consequent increase of circulation throughout the area.

There is an increase in the metabolic activity due to the increased blood supply.

The effect on the sensory nerve endings is one of analgesia, or reduction in pain; the pain reduction helps to reduce spasm present in underlying muscle tissue.

Warmth, whether it be from lamps or from some other source such as the sun, gives a feeling of general comfort and relaxation.

Radiant heat

A great number of stables have radiant heat lamps suspended from the roof or ceiling. The air flow through most stables is constant and the lamps are generally hung too high to have very much effect, particularly if the horse is rugged. The type of lamp mounted on a frame and which can be lowered so the heat source is approximately two feet away from the tissue to be treated produces the best results. Obviously, care must be taken with a horse that is tied, as excessive heat may cause skin blistering. All heat lamps should be covered by a grill to ensure that there is no possibility of the animal moving and touching the heat source.

The solarium

The solarium (Plate 5) consists of a series of infra red and ultra violet, or artificial sunlight, lamps mounted on a cradle suspended from the ceiling or roof beams. The majority of cradles can be raised and lowered, the horse standing directly beneath the lights. A set of stocks ensures that the animal cannot move and will derive full benefit of either sunlight or heat. The effects of radiant heat are identical to those produced by the single infra red lamps.

Care should be taken if a horse has stood under a solarium, and the infra red employed, for a length of time. After three quarters of an hour, the capillary dilatation may be sufficient to cause – albeit minor – a temporary fall in the blood pressure. For this reason, an animal should be allowed, after a treatment session, to rest in his box for at least an hour before being worked.

The effects of ultra violet light

Ultra violet light is a source of artificial sunlight. All living tissue benefits from controlled exposure to the sun's rays.

The amount of sunlight available to the boxed horse is reduced to exposure on exercise, and then only if the sun is out. A source of artificial sunlight can be utilised to improve the general health of animals denied the natural source.

Uses of the infra red lamps and the solarium

- To help to reduce stiffness after excessive work, i.e. competition or racing.
- To assist in the relief of pain after injury, especially after injury to the back.
- To warm a horse after an attack of colic or after typing-up.
- To dry off a horse after exercise.
- To improve the general health – especially useful for early foals and other young stock.

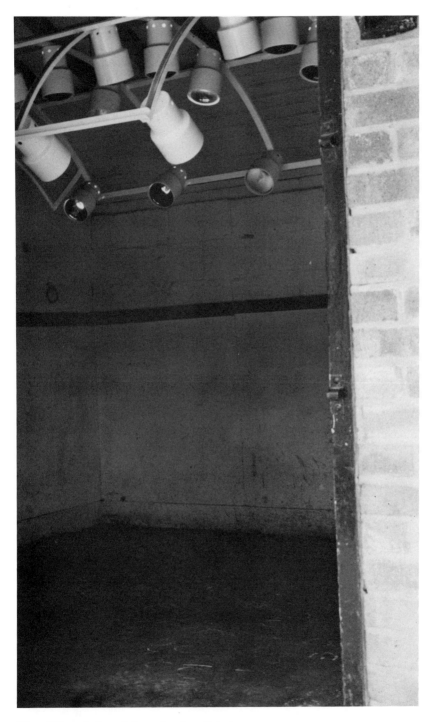

Plate 5 The solarium: infra red and sunlight lamps.

Treatment times

Radiant heat. The times of treatment depend very much upon the condition. A maximum of 30 minutes is usual for radiant heat supplied from a solarium. The lights are usually left on continuously (the radiant heat source is in the box and suspended from the ceiling).

Solarium heat can be utilised at least twice a day.

Ultra violet or artificial sunlight. It is advisable to start with a three minute exposure and to increase, over a period of 2–3 weeks, to a maximum of 15 minutes' exposure. The time of exposure may also depend upon the make of the machine – most have comprehensive instructions booklets. It is inadvisable to disregard the instructions provided. The dosage times have all been calculated by experts to ensure the best possible benefits.

Deep heat

Short wave diathermy

Short wave diathermy heats by means of a high frequency alternating current passing through the tissues. The resistance provided by the differing densities of the tissues causes the greatest amount of heat to be generated in those tissues with the greatest density, i.e. bone, a very dense tissue, heats more than fat tissue. This must be remembered if using diathermy; unacceptable heating of bone causes severe pain.

The machines are mains operated, and the animal must not be left unattended. Short wave diathermy is not very suitable for use in the animal field, particularly because the distance between the electrodes, which are mounted on adjustable arms, and the skin must remain equal. The distance between skin and electrode must be similar on both sides of the body; dissimilar distance will cause uneven heating, and possibly even a burn, should the electrode/skin gap be too narrow.

Effects of short wave diathermy

The effect of heat on tissue is always similar: increase in the blood supply. Radiant heat increases the blood supply in the superficial tissues; short wave diathermy heats the deep tissues.

Uses: any injury lying deep – for example, the joints of the vertebral column.

Treatment times

15–20 minutes on alternate days.

Contra indications

- Any form of metal implant (after fracture, pinning or plating may have been used).
- Any suspicion of malignant disease.
- Recent haemorrhage in the area of injury.
- Grossly oedematous or swollen tissue.

Short wave diathermy is of far more use for the human patient than for the animal, in its present form.

Short wave diathermy machines should *only* be used by qualified personnel.

Heat and cold

Contrast bathing is a method of circulatory stimulation. The injured area is wrapped first in a hot compress, left in situ for 3–5 minutes; then a towel, wrung out in ice cold water, replaces the hot compress and is left in situ for a similar time length. The total treatment time should last for approximately 15 minutes and be repeated three times daily for up to a week.

Effects

The heat causes a dilation and the cold a constriction of the superficial blood vessels, increasing circulatory flow.

There is some evidence to suggest that the alternate dilation and constriction in the superficial vessels will have a 'knock on' effect, and cause a similar effect in the deep vessels.

Magnetic field therapy

The first mention of the therapeutic use of a magnet was made in 200 B.C. by the Greek physician Galen. Throughout the centuries, magnetic influence on living organisms has been a topic for discussion. In the mid 1950s, Dr Andrew Bassett, working at Columbia University, New York, began to investigate the electrical activity of bone. In the 1960s, his research group suggested that it was possible to influence biological systems with electrical command signals, which in their turn might activate cell function. Magnetic fields were the eventual choice for continued research.

School laboratory experiments include demonstrations which show the production of an electrical current in a wire when the wire is moved through a magnetic field. Substitute the tissues for wire, create a pulsed magnetic flow across the tissues, and an electrical signal in the *micro amperage* range results.

At the time of writing, the only proven research work has been directed at the healing of bone. From the research papers published, it is strongly suggested that differing pulses influence differing tissues. Work is in progress throughout the laboratories of the world to try to find the correct signals for each type of tissue and to ascertain the influence of these signals at cellular level. Some workers consider that artificial stimulation at cellular level may prove harmful and that indiscriminate use is unwise. There is extensive literature on the success of magnetic field therapy in the treatment of fractures and in bone associated conditions. At the time of writing a double-blind trial is underway, at the Equine Research Station at Newmarket, on the effects of pulsing magnetic fields on tendon injuries. Other researchers are looking at the effects on damaged nerve tissue.

A statement made in Italy in 1983, at the National Congress of the Italian Society of Physical Medicine and Research, is worthy of note: 'There are many who trade on general lack of critique in an uninformed medical community to promote electro-therapeutic devices, unbacked by sound scientific research. While field work with pulsing magnetic fields and even static magnetic fields appears to be producing interesting results, there are as yet no scientific studies to back the claims made by many of the manufacturers.'

Effects of magnetic field on tissue

Experiments with thermography (a method of measuring the heat in tissues caused by increased circulation) show that magnetic fields with specific pulses cause an increase in the blood circulation. The consequence of an increased circulatory flow and a more efficient oxygen uptake is increased tissue activity.

Cellular effects

The normal elecrical charge across the cell membrane is considered to have specific control on cell behaviour, influencing the ionic exchange across the membrane. It is proposed that changes in the local *ionic*

micro environment caused by electro-stimulation such as that produced by a pulsating magnetic field, may influence the cell and
redirect the energy behavioural pattern. As yet, these hypotheses
have been proved only in the case of bone; they have not yet been
proved in the case of soft tissue, but it is undeniable that the soft tissue
injuries, when exposed to magnetic field influence, appear to have an
improved ability to heal.

Machines

There are two main types of machines designed for animal use. Both
types are mains operated, one requiring that the injured area be
placed within the field which arises from circular coils mounted on an
adjustable arm. The second (Plate 6) incorporates the magnets in
leather holders, so constructed that it is possible to position them
anywhere on the body, either by strapping them around the limb (a
shoe for treatment of foot problems is available) or mounted on a rug
– the magnet holders attach with velcro straps.

Other devices are activated by rechargeable batteries incorporated
within the unit. One, a boot developed in America, is designed for the
treatment of legs; the firm have also developed a shoe for treatment of
problems within the foot. The manufacturers of these units make no
claim for soft tissue repair – they state the unit was designed for, and
the experimental field work done, on bone tissue.

A similar battery activated device has the operating unit mounted
on an adjustable roller. Leads pass from the unit to the pairs of
magnets, themselves contained in velcro fastened pads; these can be
adjusted to fit round any part of the leg or foot. When coupled
together, the pads permit treatment of the back or shoulders (Plates 7
and 8).

The final system, a magnetic foil, is so constructed as to produce a
continuous magnetic field. The foil is coated with ceramic, making a
flexible pad that can be bandaged over the area of injury. The
penetrable depth of this device is said to be 17 mm. The foil is also
available in specially constructed boots (Plate 9), knee pads and rugs.

Treatment times

Both mains operated machines have specific treatment times laid
down by the manufacturers. The settings are changeable and are
dependent on the type of injury. In the main, the treatment times are
for not less than 30 minutes, daily or on alternate days. The battery

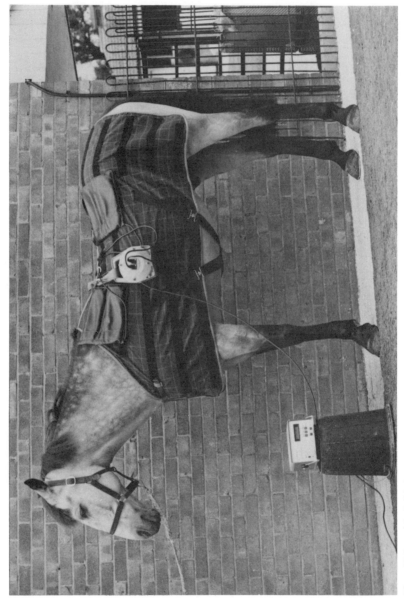

Plate 6 Magnetic field therapy.

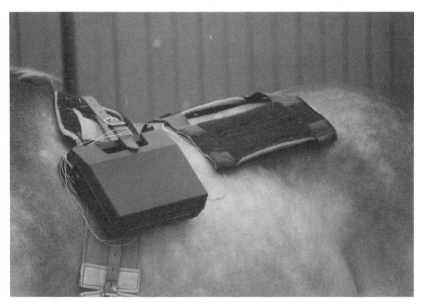

Plate 7 Rechargeable battery model.

operated machines require a minimum of two hours daily for a three week period.

The magnetic foil is placed over the damaged area and can be left on continuously – merely being removed twice daily for routine tissue checking.

Uses

Field trials unbacked by clinical trials suggest that magnetic fields influence wound healing, the reduction of post traumatic oedema, improvement in the function of arthritic joints, reduction of the pain associated with *thoraco-lumbar* problems, tendon injuries, fractures and other bone-associated conditions. While all manufacturers lay down specific treatment instructions, a minimum of three weeks' treatment is suggested even if clinical signs have disappeared. This is because, working on the hypothesis that the magnetic field has triggered cell activity by external stimuli and that the activity is not just the body's own reactive control, by the end of a 21 day period some form of effective healing should have occurred.

Field work suggests that cessation of treatment with cessation of pain (often the only objective finding), which may occur early in the treatment programme, may lead to recurrence of symptoms – in many cases with increased severity.

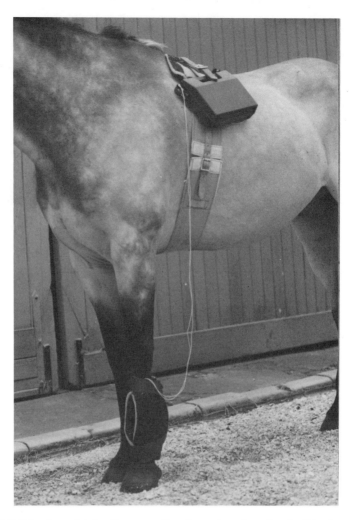

Plate 8 Felt boots containing the magnetic coils can be adapted to fit all body parts by adjustment of the velcro straps.

Contra indications

From field trials, it would appear that magnetic field therapy is *contra indicated* in any injury where there may be major damage to blood vessels. Excessive filling has occurred in some cases when magnetic field therapy has been used immediately post injury. In conjunction with a leg wash, magnetic field therapy may cause the area to blister.

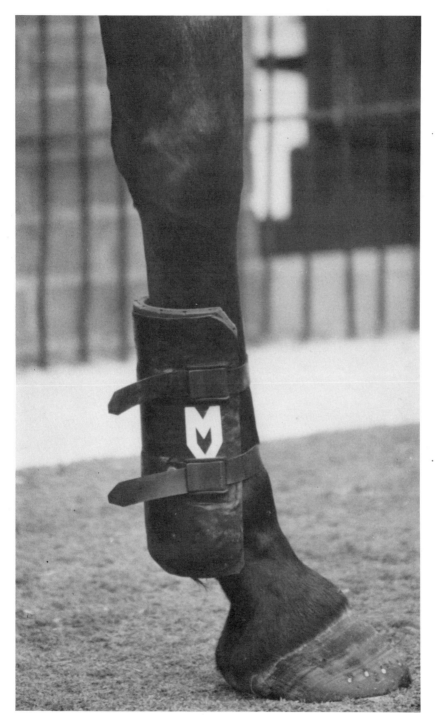

Plate 9 Magnetic field built into a boot.

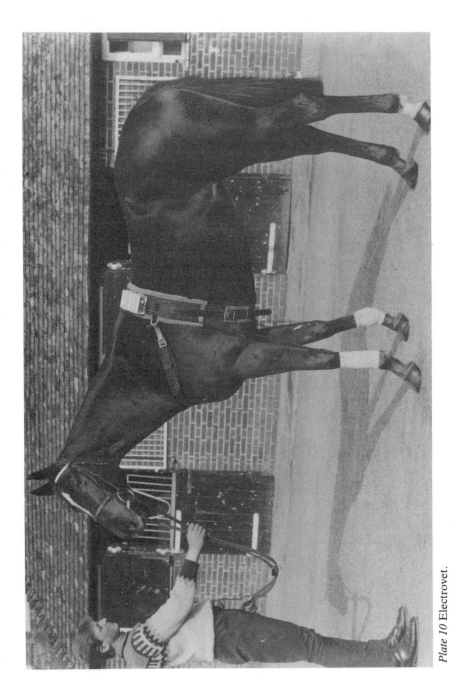

Plate 10 Electrovet.

Ionicare and Electrovet

The Ionicare unit is another recent development within the field of direct cell stimulation, so named because the type of current generated by the unit and passing through the tissues influences the ionic activity at the cell membrane.

Ions are electrically charged elements of the biological system. After injury, the ionic balance of the tissue in the area of damage is disturbed, leading to loss of function – not only of damaged cells, but also of normal cells in the area. The restoration of the balance of the intercellular ions stabilises normal cells and restores function, and also stimulates the production of materials for new cells. All these processes would occur as a normal tissue response: the current merely accelerates the start of the body's responses.

Hard on the heels of the Ionicare came the Electrovet (Plates 10 and 11). Working on the same theory, that ionic imbalance needs to be restored, but also that muscle deteriorates after injury, the Electrovet has two settings: one produces a current flow similar to the Ionicare, and the second is designed to stimulate muscle.

Both units consist of a surcingle which comprises the negative electrode, or anode. On the surcingle is mounted a pack holding a small electrical generator which is run from rechargeable batteries. The positive, or cathode, pads are applied over the area of injury and fastened in place by a small elastic bandage equipped with velcro fasteners.

The technique for using the Ionicare and the 'leg' setting of the Electrovet

The generator must be *fully charged* for effective treatment. It is wise, when using the apparatus, to see that the generator is left on charge over night; poor results are obtained if the battery within the generator is not fully charged.

The area of skin under the surcingle electrode is soaked with warm water and the towel applied to couple the electrode to the skin, which is also soaked.

The towel, folded in four, is placed just behind the withers, with the surcingle placed carefully over it and buckled firmly into place. Firm contact causes minimal skin sensation and ensures a far better treatment response by the animal. The second electrode is soaked and covered with a coupling medium or gel. The area over which this electrode will be fastened is also thoroughly soaked. This second

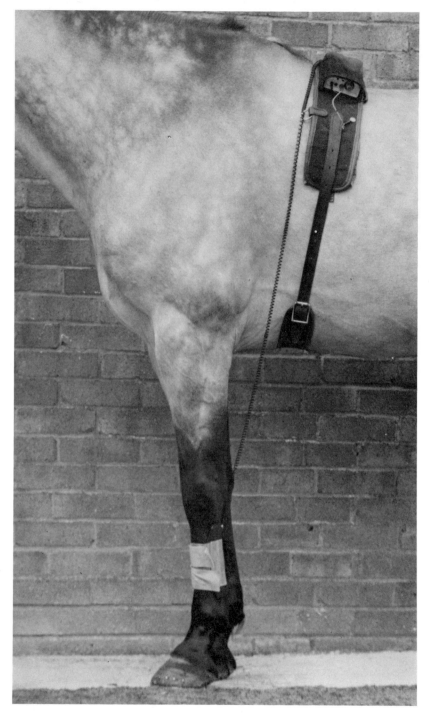

Plate 11 Electrovet.

electrode is placed carefully over and around the injured area and strapped firmly into place, either with the elastic bandages supplied or with a crepe bandage.

The leads passing from the machine to the electrodes are then attached, one end to the battery and the second clipped to the electrode itself. The final adjustment is to connect the short lead of the surcingle electrode to the generator.

The control is turned up slowly (the settings are marked from one to ten). The animal will show the current is flowing – minimal sensation will cause him to lift the leg, stamp, or twitch the underlying skin. When this occurs, the setting on the machine is turned back by at least one point.

The beauty of both devices is that they are battery, not mains, operated; the horse need not be tied during treatment but can be allowed the freedom of his box. (It is considered advisable to supply a haynet to keep the animal amused.) When treating colts or an animal that chews, it is sensible to use a bib, or even a muzzle, lest the leads be destroyed.

The unit is left in situ for up to two hours at a time. After the treatment time is completed, the machine should be turned off, the leads uncoupled, and the pads and surcingle removed. It is essential to clean the areas through which the current has passed at the end of each treatment. If this is *not* done, blistering may occur.

No current can pass into the tissues without causing a minimal skin reaction. The reaction caused by the pads of the Ionicare and Electrovet are minimal but, as treatment must be daily for a minimum of three weeks, an accumulation of salts building on the skin, under the pads, if the area is not thoroughly cleansed, will in time become an irritant.

It is advisable to wash and dry the areas, particularly if bandages need to be reapplied for support. A hair dryer is of the greatest use in this situation.

Stimulation of 'muscle' with the Electrovet

The placement of the surcingle electrode with the underlying towel is exactly similar to that utilised for the treatment of limb conditions. The small appliance at the back of the unit is changed to 'muscle' stimulation from 'leg' stimulation.

The muscle or muscles to be treated will have been identified. The area is damped and liberally covered with coupling gel.

The kit comes with large oblong treatment electrodes and smaller square electrodes. A small square electrode is the choice for muscle stimulation. The electrode must be soaked and liberally covered, on the underside, with the coupling gel. The electrode, hand-held, is placed over the muscle requiring treatment, and the intensity on the machine turned slowly up from 'O' until a muscle contraction is felt. The muscle should be allowed to contract 20 or 30 times, and then allowed a short rest before again being stimulated.

Uses:

Ionicare and 'leg' setting of Electrovet:

- Tendon damage
- Joint damage
- Local swelling after joint injury
- Windgalls
- Muscle strains

'Muscle' setting of Electrovet:

All weak muscle groups resulting from muscle strain, post traumatic atrophy or atrophy due to nerve damage.

Treatment, whether it be on the 'leg' setting or the 'muscle' setting, should be daily for a period of a minimum of three weeks.

Ultrasound

Like laser, ultrasound has more than one use in the medical field. Used for scanning, measurement, diagnosis and treatment, it is the therapeutic range that is applicable after injury. Unlike massage, muscle stimulation and heat, but as with magnetic field and laser therapy, the effects of ultrasound occur at cellular level.

Incorrectly used, it is probably the most dangerous piece of machinery on sale to the general public. Post treatment fractures, destruction of joint surfaces and deep tissue necrosis (death) have been reported in animals after treatment by unqualified personnel.

What is ultrasound?

Sound waves are pressure waves travelling through a medium such as air. They have a specific wave length, frequency and velocity. Water is a good conductor of sound; air is comparatively poor. The upper limit of hearing is just over 20 KHz (20,000 cycles per second). The therapeutic frequencies of ultrasound are well above this, being in the region of 0.75 MHz, 1 MHz or 3 MHz.

For a machine of 1 MHz, a medium that will vibrate at one million cycles per second is needed. A quartz or barium titnate crystal is used, fused to the metal plate of the transducer or treatment head. When this crystal is bombarded with a high frequency current, movement occurs in the crystal and is transmitted to the metal front plate, producing an ultrasonic wave. This wave obeys the laws of reflection and refraction.

Air will not transmit ultrasonic waves. They reflect back upon themselves and may shatter the crystal, thus the need to use a coupling medium between the treatment head and the area to be treated. The head should always be perpendicular to the surface to be treated, or refraction will occur. The measurement of ultrasound is calculated in watts/cm^2.

As the beam travels through a medium, its intensity is reduced by scattering and absorption. It has been calculated that the intensity of an ultrasonic beam decreases by a constant fraction per centimetre, known as the *half value thickness*. This depth is calculated to be 7 cm for 0.75 MHz machines, 4 cm for 1 MHz machines and 2.5 cm for 3 MHz machines. This calculable depth is of significance when treating deep structures, as the half value thickness is again reduced by half when the beam has travelled the same distance from the half value level.

It is not possible to increase the surface wattage in the hope of an increased treatment level deep down: this would harm the superficial structures. The use of a machine with the three MHz settings, their depths already described above, is the only realistic method of treating tissues of differing depth.

Machines

Ultrasound machines (Plates 12, 13, 14 and 15) are mains operated. The generator is housed in a metal box, with the control knobs on the upper surface. The controls consist of a timer, often incorporated with the on/off mechanism; a selection knob for pulsed or continuous sound; a dial which will give a read-out of the watts to the cm^2; and in those machines with more than one hertz setting, a hertz selection control.

Attached to the generator by a lead is the treatment head or transducer.

There is no way of knowing if the machine is emitting a beam other

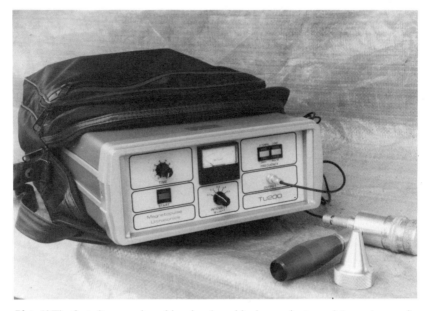

Plate 12 The first ultrasound machine developed for horses (note useful carrying case).

than by testing the machine daily. This is done either by placing the transducer in water, or by inverting the head, covering it with a treatment gel and then turning on the machine. The beam of energy is clearly visible in the water and the gel bubbles in the centre if the mchine is working.

Effects of ultrasound

These are thermal and non-thermal.

Thermal effects. These include reduction of muscle spasm, a mild inflammatory reaction including increased blood flow, and an increase in the elasticity of such structures as scar tissue.

Non-thermal effects. Research has shown that ultrasound stimulates cell behaviour and activity.

Laboratory tests on rat tissue have shown that in treated tissue there are more bundles of collagen fibres, though these bundles are finer than normal tissue, and the tissue is slightly stronger and more elastic than the tissue of the untreated control subjects. A study in Iraq (Morcos and Aswad), in 1978, on only five horses showed significant improvement in tendon repair treated with ultrasound after surgical splitting.

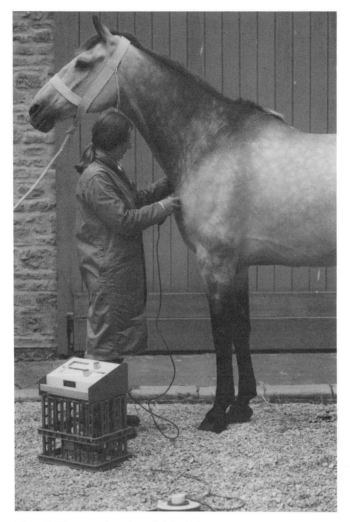

Plate 13 Ultrasound to the subdeltoid bursa.

Treatment of bone by ultrasound

Treatment of bone in the first two weeks after fracture has been shown experimentally to minimise the cartilage production phase, and shows rapid ossification, though repair in the early stages is of a juvenile-type bone. Conversely, treatment in the second stage of repair is contra-indicated, ultrasound delaying bone union by stimulating an increased production of cartilage.

The optimum time for treatment in the stimulation of bone repair

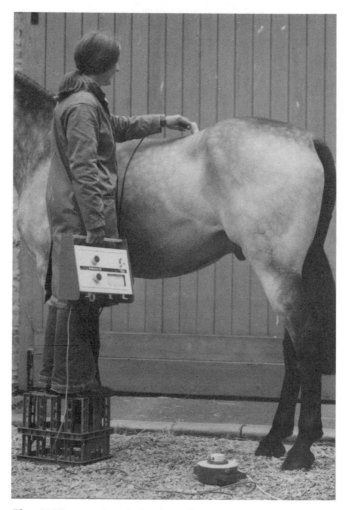

Plate 14 Ultrasound to the lumbar spine.

appears to be in weeks one and two after injury. Treatment started after this time is *not* efficacious and delays or reverses bone union.

Machines

All machines on the market were developed for the human field and have merely been renamed for veterinary use. Some are linked to muscle stimulators. The combination of ultrasound and faradic stimulation simultaneously is, in the opinion of some research workers, contra-indicated.

All machines are mains operated. The more versatile have the three

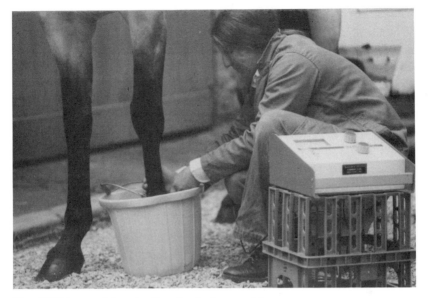

Plate 15 Ultrasound in water for a bruised sesamoid.

frequencies 0.75 MHz, 1 MHz and 3 MHz. These are the most useful, but the 1 MHz machine is the most frequently found in practice.

Treatment

Areas to be treated should be close clipped. Treatment can be given by using a coupling medium and direct contact or the immersion technique.

Contact method. A liberal supply of coupling medium should be spread over the area requiring treatment. The treatment surface of the transducer should also be lubricated. The transducer is put firmly on to the skin; the machine is timed for the length of treatment and then turned on. The intensity required is then selected. The transducer head *must* be kept moving throughout the treatment. A slow circular movement or parallel stroke movement of the head should be employed. There is some evidence to suggest that there is a better effect on tissue repair if the parallel stroke method is used, the strokes being aligned in the direction of the underlying normal tissue. Conversely, the use of a circular movement for haematoma reabsorption and the softening of old adherent scar tissue is the better (Japanese research).

Underwater method. The limb (it is only for limbs that this method is suitable) is immersed in a tub of water, e.g. a plastic dustbin. The leg must be rubbed to ensure that no air is trapped in the hair of the coat, as this air will reflect the beam away from the treatment area. The treatment head should be held parallel to the limb and approximately 1–2 cm away. Water is a good conductor of ultrasound. The head must be kept moving, as in the contact method. Remember, the lower the wattage cm/^{2}, the better the effect: *less* heat, *more* cell stimulation.

Pulsed or continuous. Pulsed ultrasound delivers two or more microseconds of sound, followed by a period of silence. The ratio of sound to rest varies with every machine. It is considered that pulsed ultrasound causes minimal heating. It is necessary to know the ratio of pulse to rest, because this is the only way that the treatment time can be calculated. In general, all treatments are given using continuous ultrasound, but the choice as to whether to use pulsed or continuous sound must be that of the operator. Severe haematomas and recent injury with massive oedema are best treated with pulsed ultrasound.

Contra indications

Avoid the brain, eyes and reproductive organs, tumors, thrombosis, heart disease, circulatory and intestinal disorders. Too high a dosage may produce periostal pain. *Always use a low output dosage.*

Do not treat if there is any suspicion of haemarthrosis or sepsis, other than sinusitus.

The treatment causes no sensation unless the dosage is too high, and is tolerated well by most horses.

Many animals are being treated over too long a period, i.e. up to three months' daily exposure. *This is harmful*, and can cause demineralisation of bone.

A month is suggested as being the maximum for a treatment regime – give at least two weeks' break before recommencing treatment.

Phonophorises

There are certain gels on the market which contain adrenocortical extracts, usually the equivalent to 20 milligrams of cortico-steroid per gram. These can be used as a coupling medium in ultrasonic therapy. As they contain anti-inflammatory and anti-exudative substances, they are of particular benefit for recent injury; this method is suggested as a non-invasive way of producing a superficial local anti-inflammatory effect.

Note: it must be remembered that cortico-steroids are banned for 14 days pre race or competition.

Laser

LASER is an acronym for the words Light Amplification by Stimulated Emission of Radiation. The concept of laser was first developed in 1916 by Albert Einstein, but the use of the low power laser is relatively new in the therapeutic field, being first used and experimented with in Europe approximately 10 years ago. It has been used in North America for the past four years.

Two general classifications of laser can be made: 'high power' or 'hot' lasers and 'low power', 'cold/soft' lasers. Hot lasers are capable of causing changes in the material irradiated as a result of excessive heat. Many people associate lasers with this, when they can be described as a 'scalpel of light' with the power to destroy, cut and coagulate tissue – an effective surgical tool.

Low power or soft lasers do not destroy. The helium neon laser (Plate 16) and the galium arsenide laser are two types produced for therapeutic use. The galium arsenide laser is usually known as an infra red laser. The effects of both the helium neon and the infra red laser appear to be similar, though a greater depth of penetration is claimed for the galium arsenide models. They are named after their active medium – that is, the medium which produces the light source. In the case of the infra red laser, this is a solid source; in the case of the helium neon, it is a gas source.

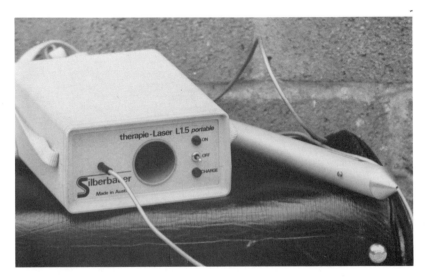

Plate 16 Helium neon portable laser.

The effect of laser irradiation on the tissues

The production of collagen is the base requirement for tissue healing. Laboratory experiments reveal that both the helium neon and infra red lasers accelerate collagen synthesis, thus assisting the acceleration of healing.

The second effect of laser irradiation is a reduction in pain, particularly if the acupuncture points are stimulated.

Laser acupuncture

In order to practice acupuncture in the traditional Chinese manner with needles, a specialist training is required. Acupuncture using the soft laser dispenses with the need to learn to insert needles, the only necessity for laser acupuncture being a knowledge of the location of the acupuncture points and – most important – to which areas and structures the differing points apply. Treatment by acupuncture is completely ineffective unless the correct points are used.

There are a wide variety of machines available for acupuncture, one of the most useful being a machine with a sensor mounted on the tip of the acupuncture probe. This sensor is capable of measuring the electrical skin resistance. The skin resistance is lower over the acupuncture points; the bleep of the sensor changes significantly, determining the presence of an acupuncture point.

To stimulate the point, the probe is held over the detected area and the laser beam activated. Some machines require as little as 15 seconds' exposure to be effective. It may be necessary to treat as many as 20 or 30 acupuncture points in order to give pain relief. The pain relief can last for as long as 10 days.

Treatment for pain, by acupuncture, is normally given once a week.

Note: the beam of a laser should *never* be directed towards the naked eye. Some makes of machine require both operator and patient to wear dark glasses.

Treatment of soft tissue by lasers

The simplest explanation of the effect of the soft laser on tissue can be summarised by stating: 'The beam of monochromatic light emitted by the laser apparatus penetrates into the tissues where it is absorbed by cells and converted into energy, influencing the processes of metabolism.'

In an area of injury, the repair processes are therefore enhanced by the extra cellular energy. As with all new technology, the claims of the effects of the therapeutic laser range across the entire spectrum of injury and disease. Many of the claims are without foundation.

Responsible field work within the veterinary sphere, done in Australia by Dr Arthur Pearce, B.V.Sc., in 1982, suggests that laser therapy was useful in the following groups of injuries:

- Tendon and ligament injuries
- Superficial joint and bone injuries
- Open and post surgical wounds
- Old fibrous injuries

The benefits of using a laser are:

(1) It is non-invasive.
(2) There is no sensation associated with the beam.
(3) There is an obvious reduction in recovery time.

It must be noted that the effect of laser therapy is still a research activity, and the implications of this sphere of treatment have not yet been fully investigated.

Open wounds

The effect of the cold laser is to accelerate wound healing, apparently without the production of proud flesh.

The laser depresses the rate of bacterial division and, as such, assists in keeping the wound sterile.

Treatment should be given around the periphery and in the centre of the crater of the wound.

Care must be taken that the periphery does not grow in, leaving pockets which may retain fluid and become infected.

As with all types of treatment, laser therapy requires skill and knowledge.

Helium neon and infra red lasers – operational hints

(1) Apply laser therapy as *first* treatment.
(2) Direct the laser beam perpendicularly to the area requiring treatment.
(3) Remember that pulsed laser is said to control pain; continuous beams are suggested for healing. You can alternate pulsed-to-continuous irradiation during each session if your machine has this facility.
(4) Leave a 2–4 day interval between sessions.

Pain aggravation may be observed after early sessions. This is a physiologic reaction – but better advise client.

Avoid combining laser treatment with anti-inflammatory drugs. Use only antibiotic coverage, if necessary.

It is advisable to shave the points/areas under treatment.

The depth within tissues to which a cold laser penetrates and is effective varies with the wavelength of the emitted beam frequency of the machine. For practical purposes, the majority of machines are effective to a depth of 10–15 mm in soft tissue.

Electrical stimulation of muscle

Muscle contraction can be mechanically achieved by stimulation via the motor nerves using a faradic current or an interrupted direct current. The latter is the choice of necessity where the nerve supply to the muscle is interrupted, for while a faradic current can produce contraction in muscle to which the nerve supply is lost, the strength of the stimuli required would be intolerable to the subject. Muscle activity cannot take place without the back up of all other body mechanisms. The body cannot move without muscle activity. Movement influences every system, and it is of prime importance to maintain muscle capability after injury.

Muscle atrophy

Muscle atrophy and weakness occurs as a result of direct injury to muscle or tendon, disuse as a result of fracture, injury to a joint, injury to partner muscle groups, and interference with the nerve supply to muscle.

Effects of electrical stimulation of muscle following injury

(1) Improves the venous and lymphatic drainage.
(2) Assists in preventing gross muscle atrophy.
(3) Prevents the formation of unwanted adhesions.
(4) Scar tissue formation is reduced to a minimum due to the maintenance of muscle mobility.
(5) Damaged or weakened muscle can be partly rebuilt and re-educated.

Muscle stimulators

There are a number of machines on the market. None – other than that developed by Sir Charles Strong, the Transeva – is specifically designed with animals in mind.

Battery operated machines are preferable to those run from mains electricity. Those designed to be strapped to the operator's waist are infinitely preferable to those that are free standing (Plate 17).

The controls mounted on the machine adjust the strength of the electrical stimulus (intensity) and the length of time the muscle remains in a state of contraction (surge).

Leads attached to *electrodes* (two in number, the *active* and the *indifferent*) are fed, by means of metal pins, into the machine. The electrodes are usually made from a thin pliable metal. They should *never* be placed in direct contact with the skin; padding, such as a lint or sponge, must lie between the skin and the metal. Direct contact can cause a skin reaction due to the chemical changes which the current flow causes in the metal.

A recent innovation is a machine about the size of a small transistor radio which can be strapped to a roller. The leads carry the current to self-adherent pads which are placed over the muscle needing to be stimulated (Plate 18). The machine is adjusted to produce the strength and length of stimulus required. When the horse has relaxed and is comfortable, and provided that a member of staff is within earshot, it is possible to leave the horse loose in the box for the duration of

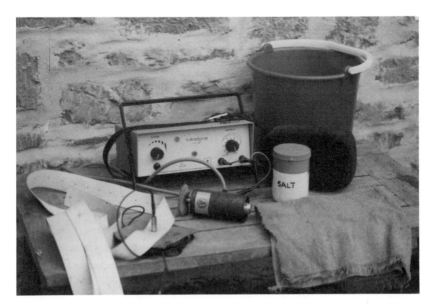

Plate 17 Faradic stimulator and accessories.

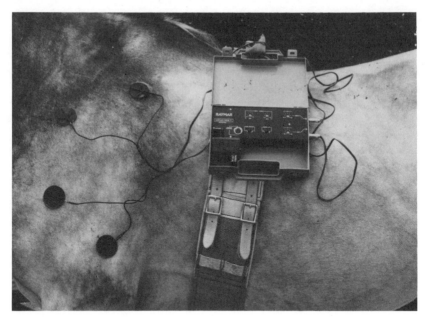

Plate 18 Horse wearing self-adherent pads on shoulder: direct muscle stimulation to shoulder.

treatment. Should a pad detach, a small bleep signal occurs which is clearly audible to people in the vicinity.

Technique of muscle stimulation

Conduction will only occur with wet electrodes and a wet coat, and saline solution is a better conductor than plain water. Make up a weak saline solution in a bucket and soak the pads you will use in the solution. Thoroughly wet the horse's coat in the area over which the indifferent electrode is to be strapped; wet the area over the muscle that requires treatment. A coupling gel or cream spread over the area allows the active electrodes to be moved freely across the coat.

The most convenient place to strap the indifferent electrode is just behind the withers. Firm contact ensures minimal discomfort as the current passes into the tissues. Ensure that the pad fits closely to the shape of the back, and girth the roller tightly. Strap the machine around your waist and make certain that all systems are at zero. Attach the lead from the indifferent pad to the machine, and then attach the lead from the active electrode, which you will hold in your hand, to the machine. Place the active electrode over the motor point of the muscle that requires treatment. (See Plates 19, 20 and 21.)

The motor point is the place where the motor nerve enters the muscle and breaks down into a series of smaller nerves. Stimulation at this point ensures the most effective muscle contraction. For approximate motor points, see Figs 13–16/Plates 22–28.

After placing the active electrode firmly over the motor point, turn on the machine; leaving the surge at zero, slowly turn up the intensity until a muscle contraction occurs. Decide if you require a quick contraction or a low contraction, and adjust the surge. Stimulate the muscle 20–30 times and then, by sliding the electrode over the dampened skin, pick up the next muscle in the group. If you are only treating one muscle, you must turn off the machine and allow the muscle a rest period before renewing stimulation. The length of the

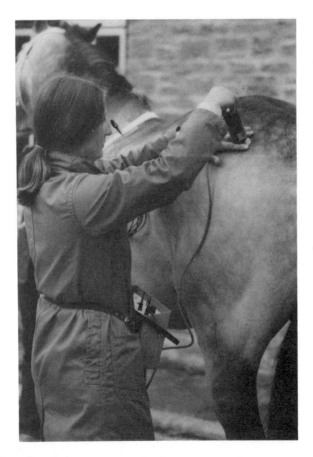

Plate 19 Faradic technique muscle-testing biceps femoris muscle. It is difficult for an unskilled operator to find motor points, lubricate the whole area and move the electrode over the surface; this will produce contraction of the entire muscle group. This method is adequate for rehabilitation but not for accurate diagnosis.

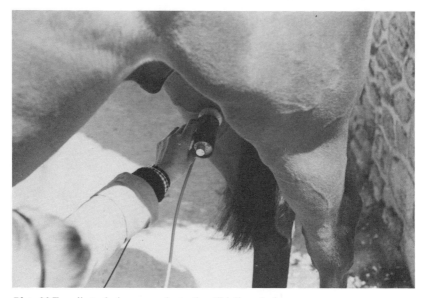

Plate 20 Faradic technique muscle-testing tibialis anterior.

rest periods are determined by the state of the muscle, the reaction of the patient and the type of injury. It is impossible to lay down fixed ruling: experience will tell you.

Diagnostic muscle stimulation

The apparatus is set up as for a treatment, but in order to use a stimulator diagnostically, the muscle reaction on the injured side must be compared to the muscle reaction on the uninjured side. Accurate readings as to the strength of stimulus required to produce a minimal contraction must be noted (the weak muscles will require a stronger stimulus).

In order to practice diagnostic muscle stimulation, a very precise knowledge of muscles, their function and motor points is required.

Stimulation of injured muscle will usually produce an adverse reaction, the horse moving away, flinching, or showing signs of discomfort.

Machines designed to give a digital reading of muscle activity are in the experimental stage, employing self adherent electrodes similar to those used in an ECG (electrocardiograph) machine (see Plate 29). Unlike the early EMG (electromyograph) machine, they are to be non-invasive – early EMG machines required the insertion of needles through the tissue to get an accurate reading. The new machines will be

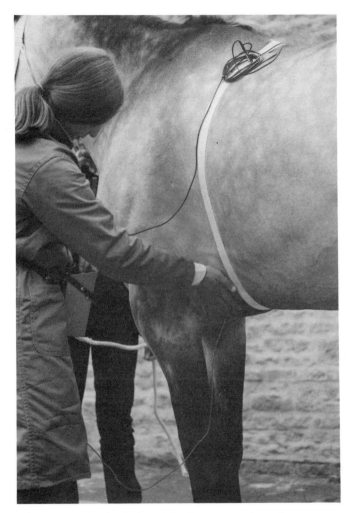

Plate 21 Faradic stimulation of the deep pectoral muscle.

commercially available within the next two to three years, for as the human field progresses, so will the veterinary field benefit.

Interrupted direct current

When the nerve supply to muscle is impaired, the muscle reacts better to an interrupted direct current passing through the tissues. The response of muscle will be sluggish. IDC can be used as a diagnostic aid to determine the extent of the loss of nerve conduction.

Due to the stimulation of sensory nerve endings and the fact that the impulses are of long duration, often giving rise to a stabbing sensation,

94

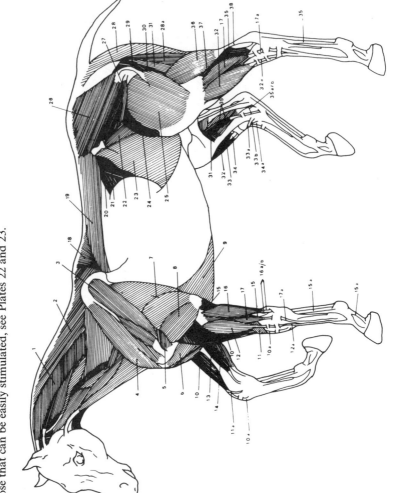

Fig. 13 Deep muscles: lateral view.

Muscles sited under the superficial layer. For those that can be easily stimulated, see Plates 22 and 23.

1. Part of semispinalis capitis; 2. Rhomboid; 3. Infraspinatus; 4. Supraspinatus; 5. Teres minor; 6. Biceps brachii; 7/8. Long and lateral head of triceps; 9. Posterior part of the deep pectoral; 10/10a. Extensor carpi radialis/see Fig. 14 Superficial muscles; 11/11a. Extensor carpi obliqus/see Fig. 14 Superficial muscles; 12/12a. Extensor digitorum communis/see Fig. 14 Superficial muscles; 13. Flexor carpi radialis; 14. Flexor carpi ulnaris; 15/15a. Flexor digitorum profundus/see Fig. 14 Superficial muscles; 16. Ulnaris lateralis; 17/17a. Extensor lateralis; 18. Thoracic part of semispinalis; 19. Longissimus; 20. Retractor costae; 21. External abdominal oblique; 22. Iliacus; 23. Internal abdominal oblique; 24. Rectus femoris; 25. Vastus lateralis; 26. Gluteus medius; 27. Deep gluteal muscle; 28/28a. Semitendinosus/ see Fig. 14 Superficial muscles; 29. Quadratus femoric; 30. Adductor femoris; 31. Popliteus; 32/32a. Extensor digitorum longus and tendon; 33a/33b. Tibialis anterior and tendon; 34/34a. Peroneus tertius and tendon; 35a/35b. Flexor digitorum profundus; 36. Gastrocnemius (lateral head); 37. Soleus; 38. Achilles tendon.

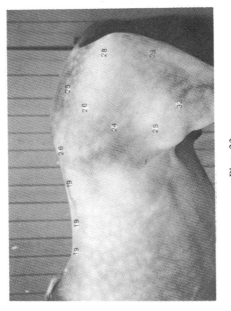

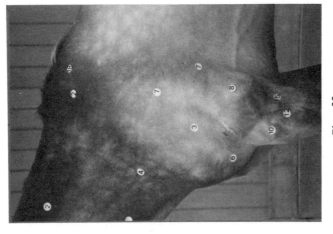

Plate 22 Motor points for muscle stimulation; 2. Rhomboid – stimulate after neck or wither problems; 3. Infraspinatus – stimulate after neck, shoulder and leg problems; 4. Supraspinatus – stimulate after neck, shoulder and leg problems; 6. Biceps brachii – stimulate after elbow or leg problems; 7/8. Long and lateral head of triceps – stimulate after shoulder and leg problems, and after radial palsy; 10. Extensor carpi radialis – stimulate after shoulder and leg problems; 12. Extensor digitorum communis – stimulate after shoulder and knee problems.

Plate 23 Motor points for muscle stimulation; 15. Flextor digitorum profundus – stimulate after leg problems; 18. Thoracic part of semispinalis – stimulate after wither problems; 19. Longissimus – stimulate after all back and pelvic problems; 24. Rectus femoris – stimulate after hip, hock or stifle problems; 25. Vastus lateralis – stimulate after hip, hock or stifle problems; 26. Gluteus medius – stimulate after all back, pelvic and hip problems; 28. Semitendinosus – stimulate after problems in hip or hock or tear in muscle; 32. Extensor digitorum longus and tendon – stimulate after leg problems.

Plate 23

Plate 22

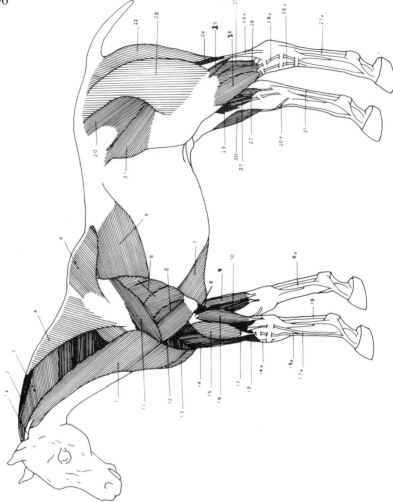

Fig. 14. Superficial muscles.
For points for stimulation, see Plates 24–26.
1/1a. Brachiocephalic muscle and tendon; 2. Rhomboideus cervicis; 3. Splenius; 4. Trapezius; 5. Latissimus dorsi; 6. Triceps; 7. Deep pectoral; 8/8a. Flexor carpi ulnaris; 10. Flexor carpi radialis; 11. Deltoid; 12. Brachialis; 13. Pectoral muscle; 14. Extensor carpi radialis; 15. Extensor digitorum; 16. Extensor carpi ulnaris; 17. Extensor digitorum lateralis; 18. Extensor carpi obliquus; 19. Superficial flexor tendon; 20. Superficial gluteal muscle; 21. Tensor fasciae latae; 22. Semitendinosus; 23. Biceps femoris; 24/24a. Gastrocnemius; 25. Soleus; 26/26a. Extensor digitorum longus; 27/27a. Flexor digitorum profundus; 28/28a. Extensor digitorum lateralis; 29. Popliteus; 30/30a. Tibialis anterior; 31. Superficial digital flexor tendon.

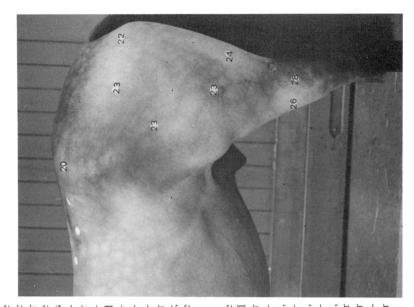

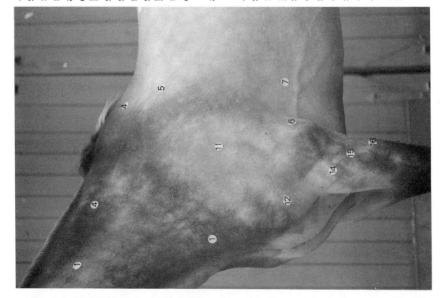

Plate 24 (left) Motor points for muscle stimulation. 1/1a. Brachiocephalic muscle and tendon – stimulate after neck problems; 4. Trapezius – stimulate after shoulder problems; 5. Latissimus dorsi – stimulate after shoulder problems; 11. Deltoid – stimulate after shoulder problems; 12. Brachialis – stimulate after shoulder problems and radial palsy; 13. Pectoral muscle – stimulate after shoulder or leg problems; 14. Extensor carpi radialis – stimulate after radial palsy; 15. Extensor digitorum – stimulate after radial palsy; 16. Extensor carpi ulnaris – stimulate after radial palsy.

Plate 25 (right) Motor points for muscle stimulation. 20. Superficial gluteal muscle – stimulate after any back or pelvic problem; 22. Semitendinosus – stimulate after problem in hip or hock, or tear in muscle; 23. Biceps femoris – stimulate after problems in hip or hock, or tear in muscle; 24. Gastrocnemius – stimulate after problems in hip or hock, or tear in muscle; 26/26a. Extensor digitorum longus – stimulate after problem in stifle joint; 28/28a. Extensor digitorum lateralis – stimulate after hip or hock problems.

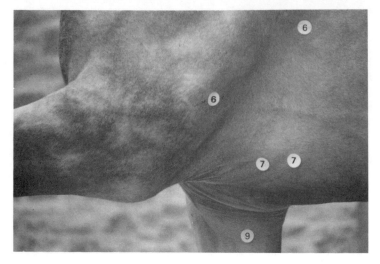

Plate 26 Motor points for muscle stimulation. 6. Triceps – stimulate after shoulder, elbow or leg problems and after radial palsy; 7. Deep pectoral – stimulate after shoulder, elbow or leg problems; 9. Flexor carpi ulnaris – stimulate after shoulder, elbow or leg problems.

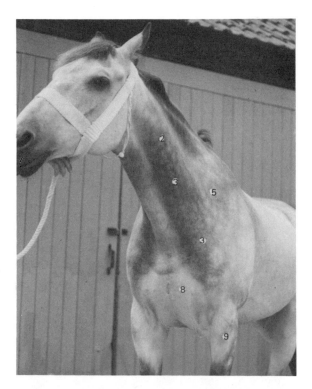

Plate 27 Motor points for muscle stimulation. 2. Sternocephalic – stimulate after neck problems; 3. Brachiocephalic – stimulate after neck or shoulder problems; 5. Supraspinatus – stimulate after shoulder or elbow problems; 8. Superficial pectoral – stimulate after any shoulder problem; 9. Extensor carpi radialis – stimulate after shoulder problems or radial palsy.

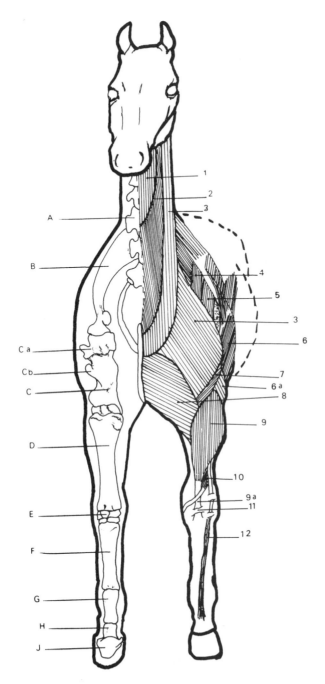

Fig. 15 Skeleton and muscles: anterior aspect. For stimulation points, see Plate 27.
Muscles: 1. Sternothryohyoid; 2. Sternocephalic; 3. Brachiocephalic; 4. Deep pectoral muscle; 5. Supraspinatus; 6. Long and lateral head of triceps; 7. Brachialis; 8. Superficial pectoral; 9. Extensor carpi radialis; 10. Extensor carpi obliquus; 11. Annular ligament; 12. Common digital extensor tendon.
Skeletal landmarks: A. Cervical vertebrae (neck); B. Scapula (shoulder blade); C(a). Point of shoulder; C(b). Upper end of tuberosity or humerus; D. Radius; E. Carpal joint (knee); F. Cannon bone; G. Long pastern (1st phalanx); H. Short pastern (2nd phalanx); J. Pedal (3rd phalanx).

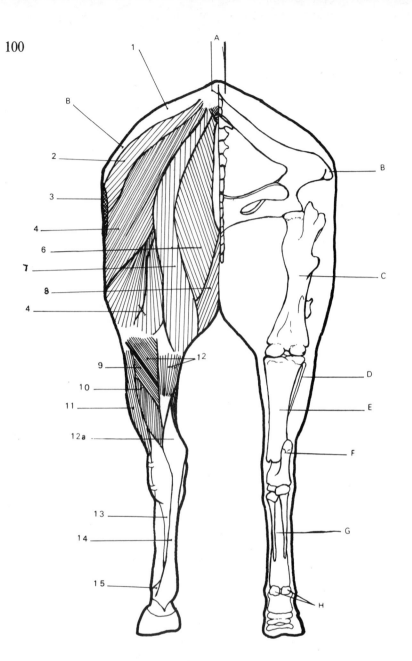

Fig. 16 Skeleton and muscles: posterior aspect. For stimulation points, see Plate 28. Muscles: 1. Gluteal fascia; 2. Superficial gluteal muscle; 3. Tensor fascia latae; 4. Biceps femoris; 6. Semitendinosus; 7. Semimembranosus; 8. Gracilis; 9. Soleus; 10. Flexor digitorum profundus; 11. Extensor digitorum lateralis; 12. Gastrocnemius; 13. Part of the deep flexor tendon; 14. Superficial flexor tendon; 15. Lateral part of the suspensory ligament.

Skeletal landmarks: A. Tuber sacrale (jumpers bar); B. Tuber coxae (point of hip; incorrectly named – the hip joint is lower); C. Femur; D. Fibula; E. Tibia; F. Point of hock; G. Cannon bone; H. Sesamoids.

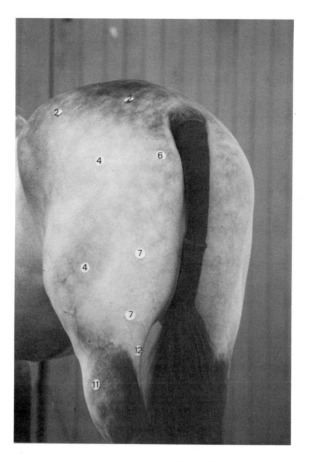

Plate 28 Motor points for muscle stimulation. 2. Superficial gluteal muscle – stimulate after problems in the lumbar spine or pelvis; 4. Biceps femoris – stimulate after problems in hip or hock, or tear in muscle; 6. Semitendinosus – stimulate after problems in hip or hock, or tear in muscle; 7. Semimembranosus – stimulate after problems in hip or hock, or tear in muscle; 11. Extensor digitorum lateralis – stimulate after stifle problems; 12. Gastocnemius – stimulate after problems in hip or hock.

this method of muscle stimulation is not satisfactory in veterinary fields. The method is mentioned only because it is still employed in some physical therapy units.

Manipulation

There are many who claim it is possible to manipulate the spine of the horse, and there are many who claim it is impossible.

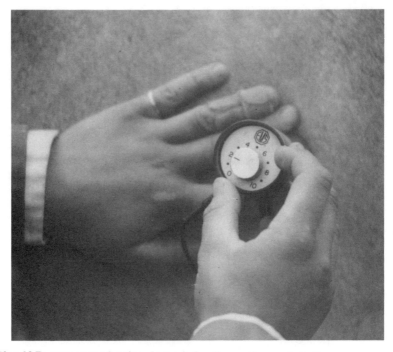

Plate 29 Remote control active electrode for diagnostic muscle testing.

Incorrect alignment of adjacent bone surfaces causes the 'computer' in the joint between those bones to record anatomical mal-
alignment; the area is not balanced as it should be, and reflex muscle
spasm results. This prevents the surfaces returning to their anatomical
normal. Even if the adjacent surfaces are only marginally out of
alignment, the imbalance is enough to stretch the supporting ligaments and cause pain.

The most reasonable explanation for the effects of manipulation are
that, having palpated, examined and discovered the area of greatest
tension in the back, the manipulator, working on the side opposite to
that of greatest tensions, strikes the muscles with a severe glancing
blow. Given with adequate severity, this will cause the muscles at the
point of impact to contract sharply, and a reflex relaxation will occur
simultaneously in their opposing group.

In a case of a minor movement of one vertebral component part on
another, the sudden relaxation of a muscle, previously in severe
spasm, could be sufficient to allow anatomical re-alignment of the
vertebral complex. Unless, however, the sets of muscles supporting
the back are in balance and of equal strength, the problem,
temporarily 'cured', will always recur.

Corrective muscle stimulation must be started immediately after manipulation, but if there is severe muscle wasting it is more sensible to build the weak muscle before attempting manipulation, lest the muscle incompetence be so great that there is no hope of retaining the correct joint alignment.

Interferential therapy

Interferential therapy is a form of electrical treatment in which two medium frequency currents are utilised in such a way as to produce a low frequency effect.

Skin has a high impedence, or resistance to current flow. In some cases, the current required to effect a treatment response could cause too much sensation within the skin tissue, making the treatment uncomfortable to such a degree that it would not be tolerable.

The apparatus consists of a mains operated generator and four pads coupled to the generator, the current passing through the tissues by means of the electrodes at the distal end of leads.

The electrodes must be placed in such a way that the two currents generated cross each other at right angles, and the tissue to be treated is in the centre of the cross of the passage of the current. While this is relatively easy to determine in the human, it is more difficult in the animal, due to the inability to discuss the actual site of pain.

People using interferential therapy within the field of animal treatment have claimed excellent results. The main advantage of the treatment is that it is possible to treat deep tissue damage. Most of the other machines on the market affect only superficial tissue.

The interferential unit should only be used by an expert; therefore discussion as to its uses is not appropriate here.

6 Rehabilitation

The machine phase is only the first part of treatment. The machines and active rehabilitation should, ideally, go hand in hand. Machines aid tissue repair, maintain and re-educate injured muscle and relieve pain, but are not a substitute for natural exercise.

Rest versus activity is a very controversial subject. Laboratory work on injured bone, muscle and tendon tissue in the rat has shown that early *controlled activity* of the injured area stimulates and assists repair; the formation of adhesions is reduced to a minimum, joint mobility is retained and full function is restored at an earlier date than in similarly injured control subjects, for whom immobilisation and rest were employed.

Most horses are turned away for rest following injury. Effective rehabilitation *before* the rest period will ensure that, when brought up to start back in work, the horse will be able to function correctly and in balance.

Injury of an acute and sudden onset is easily recognised. It is the small problems, which often pass undetected for long periods, that result in an imbalance of movement, a reluctance to lead on a certain leg, stiffness to one side, shortening of stride length, and so on. Dr Erickson of Kansas State University, using a heart rate computer, found that musculoskeletal injuries were detected, and therefore present, between 8 and 30 days prior to the appearance of obvious clinical symptoms.

The pain caused by the injury and the loss of full function of the affected areas, causing the horse to work in an imbalanced manner, also establishes a new reflex movement pattern. The cessation of pain, as a result of the machine phase of treatment, along with an improvement of the muscle tone of the injured area, cannot change the newly established reflex movement pattern. Only specialist exercise routines, designed to re-educate and produce the correct way of going, will return the horse to full potential.

If the necessary retraining cannot be instigated before the 'rest' period when the animal is turned away, the animal will still work out of balance and injury will tend to recur on resumption of training.

Swimming pool therapy

Swimming has become increasingly accepted as an adjunct to the standard methods of conditioning. The action develops excellent muscle tone, and the physical exertion helps to develop cardio-vascular function while keeping weight off the legs and joints. The majority of pools are circular. Unfortunately, the water is often cloudy and it is difficult to see the movement pattern as the horse swims.

It is important to watch the limb movements if swimming is to be of use as a treatment aid or as a therapeutic exercise. The limb movements must be even and the horse must use all four legs. Swimming is not a natural occupation for horses; they become exhausted quickly. Careful note must be taken of this, for should it happen, treatment value is lost. The use of a heart rate monitor is of great value to detect exhaustion or the onset of severe stress.

It is often difficult to achieve an even swim pattern. Some horses climb, using front legs only; others roll from side to side; others use both forelegs but only one hindleg; others will not use their front legs. An uneven pattern means uneven muscle action, and consequently uneven muscle balance.

Swimming should start with a very short session – ideally for 1–2 minutes – then the horse should be taken out of the pool, and the heart rate checked. The horse should not re-enter the pool until the heart rate has returned to an acceptable normal.

Circular swimming pools should be of large diameter, as one of the problems when swimming a horse is to persuade him to breathe. Many take a breath, close their nostrils, and rarely if ever take a second breath. The reason may well be a primitive reflex: lungs full of air produce a flotation effect.

In a small pool, the horse is on a tight circle, compressing one side of the thorax and stretching the opposite side; the strong hind leg action forces the abdominal contents forward against the diaphragm. These factors all restrict the ability of the chest to expand and allow the lungs to fill with air. As swimming is a strenuous exercise, the working muscles require oxygen. Deplete the supply of oxygen by restricting the ability to breathe, and the animal becomes exhausted; the heart rate rises in response to the oxygen requirement, creating stress conditions, and the value of the exercise is lost.

Post swimming lung haemorrhage (bleeding) has been reported. Scoping, post swimming, is one of the factors that has led to the condemnation of swimming as an exercise by some critics. The reason for the breakdown of lung tissue, with consequent bleeding, could well be impaired respiration coupled with an unacceptably high heart rate.

The benefits of swimming correctly, with all four limbs working, will never replace work on the ground, but is a useful adjunct in both a rehabilitation and a training programme.

A. C. Synder, at Ball State University, examined the adaptations of bone in horses who were trained for a short period of time on a swim versus a ground work programme. It is known that physical training increases bone density, but it is not yet agreed if both muscle contraction and the effects of the high concussion of the limb meeting the ground are required to achieve these bone adaptations. The results of Synder's trial indicate that bone may well increase in density better with a swimming than with a ground work programme.

The difficulty with any training programme is to establish the correct paramaters for such a swim training regime.

Pools

A useful type of pool is the straight pool (Plate 30), the horse walking down a ramp to the swimming area, swimming through and leaving the pool via the second ramp situated at the far end of the swimming area. Underwater jets built into the sides of such a pool can be utilised to activate a current against which the horse must work. The strength of the current, varied by the number of jets used, is dependent on the fitness and capability of the animal. After sufficient exercise, the jets are turned off; the horse swims to the second ramp and leaves the pool.

Swimming can, and in the author's opinion should, be monitored with a heart recording apparatus. Not only is this a method of checking that the heart rate of the animal is not becoming unacceptably high, but also the time taken for the heart to return to normal after exercise indicates the fitness level achieved. Should the heart rate become unacceptably high, the horse must leave the pool and rest until the heart rate returns to an acceptable normal. The improvement in fitness is considerably easier to monitor by this method, and there is no possibility of unacceptable stress, which can only cause damage.

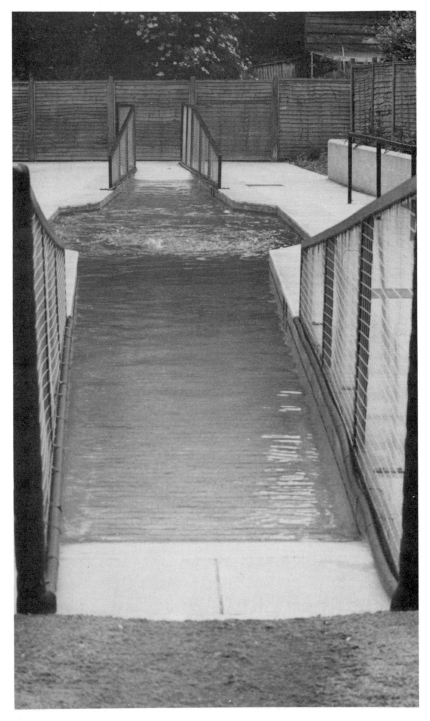

Plate 30 The straight pool.

Water walking

To re-educate muscle when a swimming pool is not available, walking in water may be used. The horses of owners living on the coast derive great benefit from wading through the sea. Streams, rivers, or lakes with sound bottoms can also be utilised for this purpose.

Some equine swimming pools have wading areas attached, and it is not difficult to construct such a useful piece of rehabilitation equipment. All that is necessary is to dig out a circular trough with approximately the same diameter as the normal 'hot walker'. The trough needs to be about 3'6" to 4' wide and a minimum of 2'6" deep. The water depth is approximately knee high. The horse is led in via an entry ramp, a gate is closed across the entry point and the horse is led round wading in the trough, the attendant walking on the ground by the side.

The resistance presented by the water improves the muscle tone of all the limbs, while the action required to lift the limbs out of the water in order to achieve forward movement is excellent for improving the tone of the muscles of the back and loins.

Water treadmills

Developed in the USA, water treadmills incorporate a moving floor as the base of the water tank. One ramp leads down to the tank base, and there is an exit ramp. After entering the tank, the horse is tethered; a bar is adjusted in front at chest height and a second bar slotted behind the quarters, these keeping the animal stable. Water is pumped slowly into the tank, the depth adjusted to achieve either partial weight bearing on the limbs when the level comes up to the belly, or full weight bearing when the water level is at either mid-cannon or above the knee.

Once the horse is accustomed to standing in the water, the motor activating the treadmill floor is started and the speed adjusted to achieve the exercise required. As with swimming therapy, it is of the greatest benefit to utilise a heart rate computer to monitor the exercise stress level and recovery rate.

The treadmill

The treadmill (Plate 31) provides the ability to exercise a horse on a non-slip surface with minimum concussion, at speeds that vary from the walk to full gallop. Most designs allow an adjustment of angle of

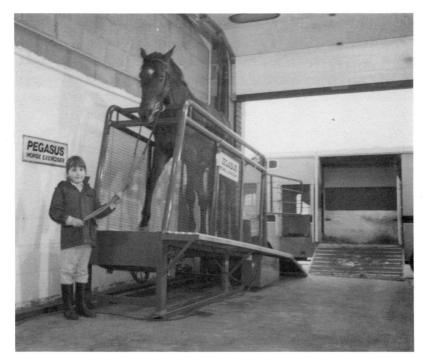

Plate 31 The treadmill.

the track, from flat to a reasonably steep incline. It has been suggested that too severe an incline may cause hock problems, and that work on a flat surface is of most benefit. The ability to exercise the muscles, particularly those of the back, by allowing them to work unhindered by either saddle or rider weight is of the greatest value.

Primarily used in Australia and America, treadmills are just beginning to be used in the United Kingdom. The majority of horses appear to take to them well, but it is necessary to introduce the exercise very cautiously. The main disadvantage of most types is that the horse has to back off the apparatus at the end of the session. This is sometimes difficult to achieve with a young animal that has never learned to back to command. Make certain you can persuade the horse to go backwards before loading him on to the apparatus.

Swimming pools, water walks and treadmills utilise all the muscle systems of the animal's body, and all are of great benefit in rehabilitation. When all systems are available, the progression should ideally be:

(1) Non weight bearing exercise in pool.

(2) Water walker or treadmill.
(3) Work on an all weather surface, the horse driven in long lines rather than being lunged on a single rein.
(4) Basic schooling – ridden.

The aims and objects of rehabilitation at the ridden phase are:

(1) To produce a flexible horse that is working in balance.
(2) To rebuild the muscle power for the task that he has to perform.

To this end, a series of gymnastic exercises can be achieved with the use of the 'BLOK' and poles. Work over poles is of enormous benefit, both to young animals and to older animals whose paces need correction. The effects depend on the arrangement of the poles. When utilised properly, light, supple, even paces with a good outline are achieved. In the case of an animal that has been injured, the pole arrangement should be adjusted to achieve even cadence. Due to the striding required to take the limbs across the layout of the poles, a correct reflex pattern of movement is re-established. (See Plates 32, 33, 34 and 35.)

Rehabilitation is a specialist subject requiring knowledge and a great deal of patience and sympathy, along with the ability to gauge just when to 'push for more'.

The horse must be comfortable in his surroundings; his tack must fit; he must not be hurt, confused or asked to work for too long at any one task. The pain of injury may still be imprinted in his memory – with

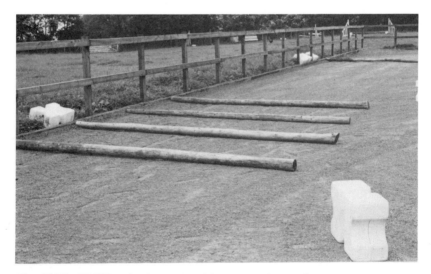

Plate 32 The BLOK and poles arranged for gymnastic exercises.

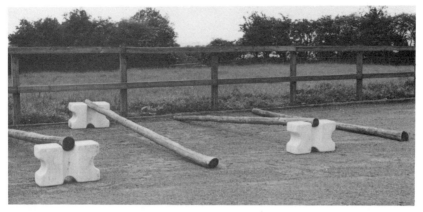

Plate 33 The BLOK and poles arranged for gymnastic exercises.

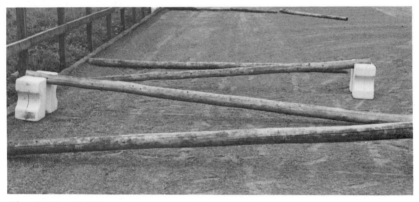

Plate 34 The BLOK and poles arranged for gymnastic exercises.

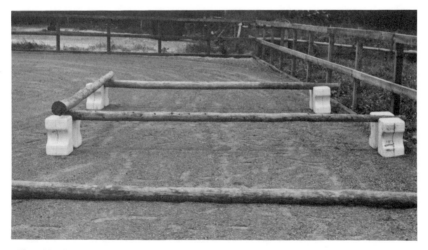

Plate 35 The BLOK and poles arranged for gymnastic exercises.

the resultant reluctance, and sometimes determination, not to perform certain tasks.

The skill of rehabilitation is to design tasks that overcome such problems without causing pain or fear.

Unfortunately, lack of time is usually the greatest factor in determining the return of an animal to its discipline. Often, rigorous training starts too early, with consequent poor results and the horse gaining a reputation for being 'ungenuine'.

As when using machines, there can be no set programmes laid down in black and white to achieve perfection after injury. Try to think how you might feel in circumstances similar to those the horse is experiencing: how bored would you be, asked the same questions again and again, if it hurt to give the answers?

The most successful horsemen and trainers are those who can relate to the animal and, by an intuitive ability, appreciate his problems – then, with tact, help and sympathy tempered by the necessity for a disciplined response, work with the animal to achieve the best possible performance.

7 The Back – Horse and Human

The discussions relating to back problems, what causes them, what cures them, and whether manipulation really works, must be the most controversial subject in the fields of veterinary and medical science.

In order to achieve any sort of understanding of the back, a mental picture of its construction and functional ability must be achieved.

The horse

The backbone of the horse consists, on average, of 54 interlocking bones or vertebrae, divided into five sections: the neck contains seven bones, the thorax or mid back eighteen (from whose bodies spring the ribs), the lumbar or loin area has six bones, the sacrum five fused together to form one block, and the tail between 15 and 21.

The construction of the vertebrae is such that movement occurs not only between the adjacent bodies of the bones, but also in small joints called *facets* or *zygapophyseal* articulations. These joints are formed by small bony extensions which project upward and outward on either side of the spine of the vertebrae, lying above the bony ring of the spinal canal and connecting with the projections from the adjacent vertebrae.

The bodies of the vertebrae are cushioned one from another by intra-vertebral discs, as in the human spine, but there is no evidence to suggest that disc damage occurs or is a primary cause of pain and malfunction of the equine spine.

The extent of movement in the spine of the horse is determined, as is the mobility of all joints, by the shape and angle of the surfaces between opposing bone ends (Plate 36).

The neck and tail of the horse possess considerable mobility, and also muscles whose function is to produce movement in these areas. Thus the horse can raise and lower his head, and turn to bite his flanks; the tail can move up and down, and swish from side to side.

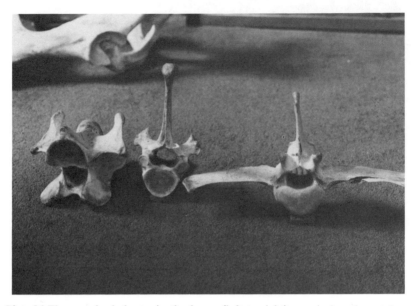

Plate 36 The vertebral shapes in the horse (left to right): cervical neck vertebra, thoracic or mid-back vertebra and lumbar vertebra.

The spine from withers to croup is remarkably inflexible. The shape and angle of the facet joints of the thoracic spine allow some up and down movement but their design allows for more side bending, while the facet joints of the lumbar spine are constructed to allow a greater degree of up and down movement than is possible in the thoracic area and little or no side flexion.

Movements of the thoraco-lumbar spine are undeniably present, and in response to pressure in specific areas, the horse can respond by performing the movements of *dorsi* or *ventro* flexion and of *side* flexion. These movements are not part of the horse's day to day activities: have you ever seen a horse stand in a field and hump and hollow his back?

The muscle groups above, below and on each side of the spine are designed to support the spine, in partnership with the abdominal muscles and three very important ligaments. The combination of the spine, ribcage and pelvis forms a tube to which are attached the limbs.

Movement of the body mass occurs as a result of, first, the forelimb being extended and fixed on the ground; secondly, the force created by the combination of a push from the rear and contractions of the muscles behind the shoulder blade slides the body mass forward, around the pivot at the upper area of the shoulder blade.

The ligaments involved (Fig. 17) work rather as do the cables of a

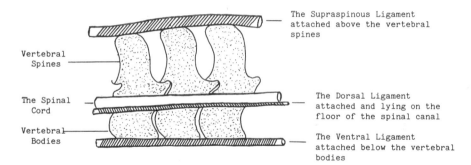

The Supraspinous Ligament
attached above the vertebral
spines

Vertebral
Spines

The Spinal
Cord

The Dorsal Ligament
attached and lying on the
floor of the spinal canal

Vertebral
Bodies

The Ventral Ligament
attached below the vertebral
bodies

Fig. 17 The ventral, dorsal and supraspinous ligaments.

suspension bridge. Three in number, they are attached to consecutive vertebrae along the length of the spine. The *ventral* ligament lies on the underside of the vertebral bodies, the *dorsal* ligament floors the tunnel of the spinal canal, and the *supraspinous* ligament – known as the nuchal ligament in the cervical area – jumps from poll to withers, sending a fan-like set of extension cables forward and down to attach to the cervical vertebrae, continuing its course attached to the spines of the thoraco-lumbar vertebrae, and ending at the sacrum (Fig. 18).

The weighty head is extremely important in assisting in the maintenance of the normal contours of the back. The ligamentum nuchae acts as a bow string between poll and withers, thus the lower the head, the tighter the bow string and the greater the traction force along the length of the spine. Raise the head, the bow string loses tension, and there is less supporting traction for the thoraco lumbar area (Fig. 19).

Many horses with 'sore' backs have been 'cured' by repositioning their head at exercise.

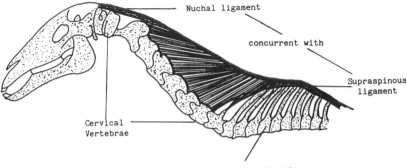

Nuchal ligament

concurrent with

Supraspinous
ligament

Cervical
Vertebrae

Thoracic Vertebrae

Fig. 18 Diagram of the nuchal ligament, showing fan-like attachments to cervical vertebrae.

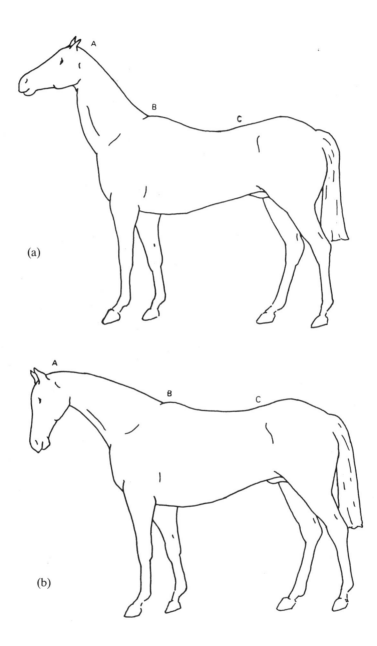

Fig. 19 (a) Head raised – distance between A and B shortens; traction on nuchal ligament reduced, strain on back at C. (b) Head lowered – distance between A and B correct; traction on nuchal and supraspinous ligament normal, back supported.

Back problems

Severe problems are very incapacitating and give rise to obvious clinical and X-ray findings. Amongst these comes the 'wobbler syndrome': the animal loses the ability to co-ordinate his movements, crossing the hind legs and 'wobbling' from side to side. The cause is pressure on the spinal cord within the canal. Other than spinal decompression – an operation to remove the pressure – little can be done.

Vertebral and pelvic fractures manifest with reluctance on the animal's part to move, and every indication of severe crippling pain associated with gross muscle wasting. Any form of treatment calls for close veterinary supervision; all cases eventually require muscle stimulation and rehabilitation.

The 'problem back' is the one producing some signs of discomfort and reduction in performance ability, but without obvious clinical findings. These types of back are almost certainly a result of ligament strain and associated muscle problems.

A disturbing feature of the aching back is the fact that the great majority of so-called 'backs' are not backs at all. Soreness and discomfort in the back has occurred as a result of a problem in a limb causing the horse to work out of balance, the uneven stresses falling on the back. The uneven stresses cause pain and the 'back experts' have a field day. The answer is to find and cure the limb problem, and then the back will recover. A recent case, seen for recurrent problems in the withers and many times manipulated, was found on examination to have a fracture of a pastern bone.

That the horse of today is subjected to stresses and strains for which it was not designed, and has not yet adapted, is well illustrated by examining the collection of spines in the Anatomy Department of the Natural History Museum in London. All the Thoroughbred spines show some form of bone damage or abnormality in the lumbar spine or lumbo sacral area; the Hackneys show spinal abnormalities at the thoraco lumbar junction; the spine of the Mongolian wild pony is perfect, as are the spines of the specimens of mules and donkeys. Examples of spinal abnormalities are illustrated in Plates 37 and 38.

The problems in the lumbo sacral area may well be explained by considering both the pivot areas of limb movement and the dissipation of the G force stresses experienced when a single limb hits the ground at fast paces. As already discussed, the G force is in the region of 350 times the horse's own body weight. At walk and trot, the front legs pivot around the upper part of the shoulder blade, and the hindlegs

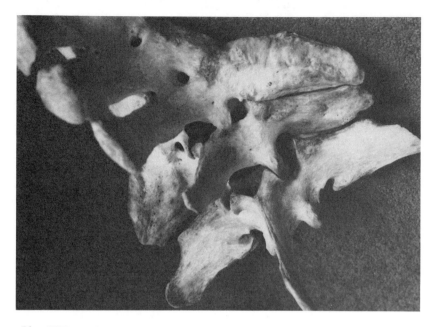

Plate 37 Bone abnormality between the last lumbar vertebra and the sacrum. Note fusion on right of picture.

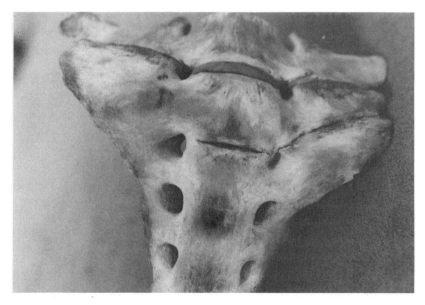

Plate 38 Reduction of diameter of aperture for the emergence of the nerve, on the opposite side to the fusion.

around the hip joint (during the gallop phase, the pivot point for the hindlegs moves to the lumbo sacral junction).

The shock waves generated as individual feet hit the ground travel up the limb involved, not as one smooth wave motion but as a series of intermittent stresses; those from the forelimbs angle backwards and terminate at the thoraco lumbar or lumbo-sacral junction – the length of the back and muscle mass of the animal determining the final location (the longer the back, the further forward the impact). The hindlimb forces travel upward through the gluteal mass, then angle forward and terminate at the fourth or sixth cervical vertebrae. The two impact energies cross in the thoraco-lumbar or lumbo-sacral area; thus at fast speeds and when jumping, all the major stresses arrive at the point of hindlimb pivot in the loins (Fig. 20).

The sacroiliac joint provides a second problem area. The 'joint' is not a true joint; no movement occurs between the two bone surfaces. It is a meeting place of two bones. Injury to the ligaments supporting the joint causes instability, with subsequent pain and loss of efficient movements of the hindlimb of the side affected.

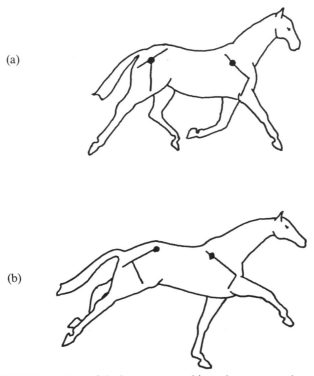

Fig. 20 (a) Pivot points of the horse at trot – hip and upper scapular areas. (b) Pivot points of the horse at gallop – lumbo sacral junction and upper scapular area.

Amongst the reasons for muscle atrophy, discussed in an earlier chapter, was the absence of an adequate nerve supply. Damage to soft tissue causes local swelling. Superficial swelling causes the skin – endowed with elastic properties – to stretch, the skin stretch relieving the pressure on the deeper structures. In areas close to the vertebral column, the swelling has no escape route.

The muscles of the back are supplied by nerves lying in and around the tissues that are damaged by excessive strain to the loins and pelvic area. The resultant swelling, in some cases, presses on the motor nerves supplying the back muscles, with subsequent temporary loss of communication to the muscle supplied by that nerve. There is immediate atrophy of muscle, with all the associated problems: loss of support for that sector of the back, loss of stability in the joints, excess strain on the ligaments that partner the muscle involved, uneven muscle balance in the area – all factors that, without treatment, will lead to continuing malfunction of the area.

To summarise, first seek the cause: it may not be in the back, especially if recurrent episodes are reported. If there is a genuine back problem, reduce the pain, stimulate the appropriate muscle groups, re-educate the movement pattern, check the saddle fit and find the cause.

Or could it be your back problem causing the horse's? An interesting case history is worth relating.

A heavy hunter, aged eight years, was admitted with back problems. On arrival, the history was of a progressive reluctance to jump, the problem becoming worse over a three year period and culminating in lameness in the near hind. Discussion provided the information that the horse always rolled excessively after exercise and was cast at least once a week, always with the near side upper most. Examination revealed gross wasting of the back muscles over the loins on the near side and some loss of the middle gluteal muscle of the near hind quarter. Back movements were grossly restricted and painful. The horse was sent for scanning; this revealed osteoarthritis of the near side hip and inflammatory changes at the lumbosacral junction.

Treatment consisted of magnetic field therapy, ultrasound, muscle stimulation and, eventually reschooling. At the end of three months, the horse was back in work, happy and pain free but reluctant to jump. The owner came to ride out before removing his horse and used his own saddle; immediately after being unsaddled the horse, in obvious pain, got down in his box to roll – something he had ceased to do. Examination of the saddle, by a saddler, disclosed a warped crooked tree.

Three years of pain, ending with an irreversible change in the hip due to the stress associated with getting cast; getting cast because the pain in his back caused him to roll, all for saddle fit. Discussion with the owner revealed he had always had back pain after riding that particular horse!

The human back

The body is balanced on the feet – superbly constructed, when they are allowed to function correctly, to absorb and dissipate the shock of meeting the ground, to propel the body forward and to record and process, through a mass of 'computers' sited on the sole, quantities of vital information. Shoes interfere badly with natural foot function, and a great deal of inbuilt perception is lost. The Zola Budds of this world train without shoes – is this the key to their success?

The ankle and knee are hinge joints, their construction and the angle of muscle pull designed to allow no rotation or turning movements.

The hip joint is a ball and socket, or universal joint; movement is possible in all directions, movement both of the body on the legs and the legs on the body.

The pelvis rests on the top or head of the upper bone of the leg, the femur. It consists of three bones joined in such a manner that there is no movement, as in other joints, but only 'give' where they meet. The sacrum, the middle bone of the three, forms the base for the spine, or vertebral column, consisting of five lumbar (low back) vertebrae, 12 thoracic (chest) vertebrae, and seven cervical (neck) vertebrae. The vertebrae are divided one from other by discs.

The structural angles of the pairs of small joints at the back of each vertebral body determine the movement possible in each area. The low back, or lumbar, area allows forward and back movement as well as side bending; rotation, or twisting, occurs mainly in the chest or thoracic area, while the neck is capable of a wide range of movement in all directions. The amount of movement between each pair of vertebrae is small. Spinal movement is achieved by the accumulation of the small movements throughout the entire vertebral column.

John Gorman, a chartered engineer, made an analysis of the human back in 1983. His findings, based on engineering principles, show that the back, used correctly, is well designed. Gorman suggests it is not the design of our backs that causes problems. Most occur as a result of stresses to which the back is subjected – put any joint through a movement range greater than it is designed to perform, and you cause damage.

He rightly pointed out that the hip joint is capable of a very large range of movement – approximately 180° – and is also the strongest joint in the body. In the western world, the way of life is such that rarely do we use more than half the available range (Fig. 21); present at birth, the wide range reduces as we fail to retain the full elastic stretch of the muscles controlling the hip joint. Because of the interrelationship between hip and back, reduce the available movement at the hip and immediately the back must endeavour to increase its movement range to comply with the action required. Damage results.

Obviously, disease causes back pain; but disease is not the subject of this text. Nevertheless, accurate diagnosis is, as always, the main requirement in any condition. Because pain in the back can be caused by a number of problems, X-ray is always advisable to determine the state of the bones. Falls can cause fractures of any part of a vertebra, leaving a temporarily unstable area. Because of the proximity of the spinal cord and nerves to the vertebral bodies, permanent damage to this vital system can occur if serious conditions are ignored.

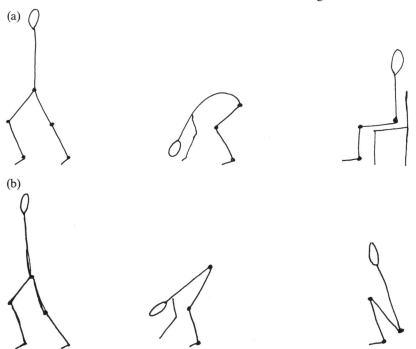

Fig. 21 The use of the hip: (a) Western man; (b) natural man.

Unless caused by disease or bony abnormalities, back pain is a soft tissue problem involving either the disc, the small joints at the back of the spine (the facet joints), the ligaments supporting the spine, or the muscles of the spine.

The discs

The discs are washers cushioned between two vertebrae – the outer wall built rather like a Radial X car tyre, strongly constructed to avoid the possibility of a 'blow out' when under normal stress. The material contained within this outer wall is rather like the material of the horse's frog. Centrally placed is the nucleus acting as a central pivot point, the effect being similar to placing a marble between two flat surfaces; one surface balances above the other and movement is possible. (See Figs 22 and 23.)

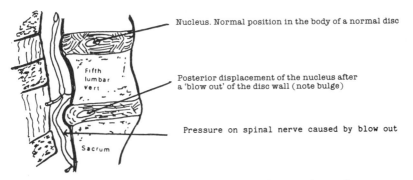

Nucleus. Normal position in the body of a normal disc

Posterior displacement of the nucleus after a 'blow out' of the disc wall (note bulge)

Pressure on spinal nerve caused by blow out

Fig. 22 Diagram of a vertical section of the fifth lumbar vertebra and sacrum.

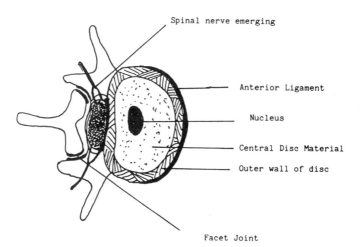

Spinal nerve emerging

Anterior Ligament

Nucleus

Central Disc Material

Outer wall of disc

Facet Joint

Fig. 23 Diagram of a cross section of a disc.

The discs can be damaged when movement stress for which they were not designed occurs – for example, bending forward and twisting, or overloading when bending forward and lifting a weight that is too heavy. Under these types of stresses, some of the fibres of the outer wall of the disc break down and a bulge appears in the area of the breakdown. Due to the position of the ligaments that hold the vertebrae together, these bulges can only occur in certain areas. Unfortunately, these areas always involve a highly sensitive nerve complex – result: pain.

Disc pain is rarely felt at the site of the problem. Nerve tissue is highly complex. An easy way to visualize the problem of pain is to appreciate that all nerve impulses travel electrically and that the reaction of nerve tissue to any unusual circumstances is to record pain. This pain is recorded in a number of ways: it may be an ache, like toothache; a continuous soreness; sudden, sharp electric shocks or twinges. Over-stimulation of a nerve creates so much electricity that the impulses discharge down the entire course of the nerve involved, their destination being determined by the path of that particular nerve; thus a severe disturbance in the low back may well cause pain to be felt down to the toes, in the neck the pain may radiate down an arm to the fingers, and in the chest the pain may be felt at the front of the chest and may make breathing uncomfortable.

Sacroiliac joint pain

The two sacroiliac joints (Plate 39) are sited at the back of the pelvis, lying just below the two dimples at the top of the buttocks. They are not true joints, just a meeting of bone to bone. Held together by immensely strong bands of ligaments, they have no muscles to move or support them; but as one bone can 'give', spring-like, against its fellow, the ligaments are subjected to over-stretch forces in certain movement conditions. Pain results, this pain usually radiating into the buttock and/or down the leg of the side affected.

Facet joint sprain

Movements occurring when the muscles and ligaments are over-strained or caught 'off guard' may sprain a facet joint (Plate 39). The joint is forced through a movement range greater than it was designed to perform, and sprained. The immediate response is local muscle spasm, loss of movement and pain. This pain may radiate from the site of injury, just as with disc problems.

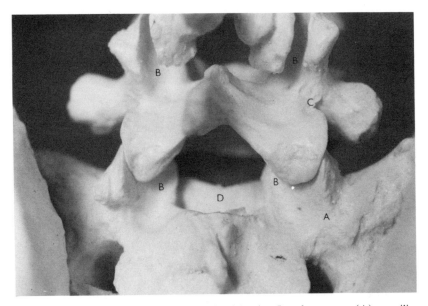

Plate 39 The human spine viewed from the back lumbar 5 on the sacrum: (A) sacroiliac joint; (B) facet joints; (C) aperture for emergence of spinal nerve; (D) canal for spinal cord.

Back muscles

Support of the back is achieved by the layers of muscles lying behind the spine working in balance with the muscles that run from the bottom of the chest to the pelvis, the abdominal muscles, and also certain of the muscles around the hip joint.

When all the muscles are in balance, the back works well. Injury always involves muscles, and after injury the back rapidly becomes out of balance. Unless this situation is corrected, the problems will always recur.

Which comes first? Do you give the horse a back, or does he give you one?

Once again, we speak of balance. The rider in perfect balance distributes weight evenly, via the saddle, to the back of the horse (see Plate 40). The horse going in balance causes an even pattern of upward thrusts to be experienced by the rider through buttocks, sacroiliac joints and back.

The moment balance is lost, things go wrong. Uneven, unequal stresses are created and damage occurs. This damage may be minimal at first, but if the situation is not corrected, endless discomfort for both horse and rider results (see Plates 41 and 42).

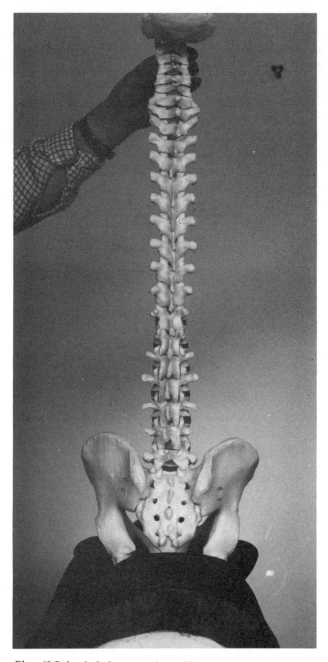

Plate 40 Spine in balance on the saddle.

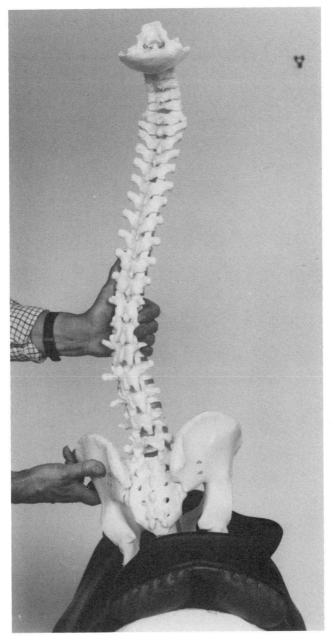

Plate 41 Left hip dropped. Note stress areas: a rotation has occurred – rider pain will be felt in low back.

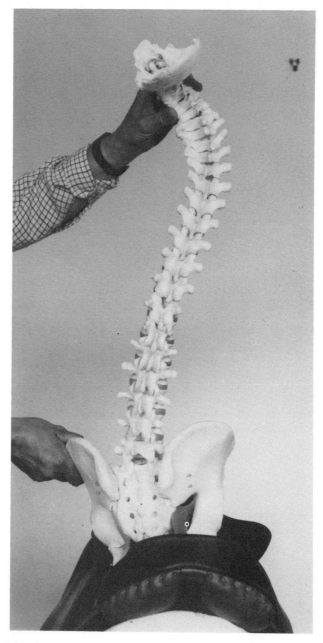

Plate 42 Left hip dropped. Note stress areas of spine: rider pain will be felt at 'bra line' and bottom of neck.

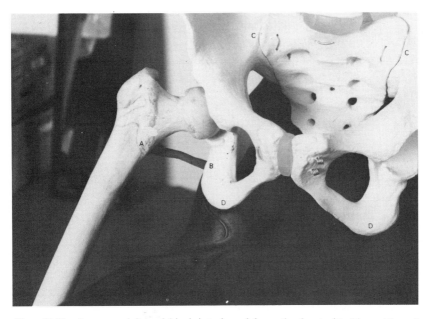

Plate 43 The human pelvis and hip joint viewed from the front: (A–B) position of adductor muscle; (C) sacroiliac joints; (D) ischial tuberosities – the bones you sit on.

In order to achieve a comfortable, secure position in the saddle, with minimal stress to the back, there must be adequate movement at the hip joints. If the adductor muscles (Plate 43) are too tight, the correct leg position is nearly impossible to achieve, balance is lost and once again there is the potential for injury.

8 Common Rider Injuries

Rider injuries

Rider injuries in the main occur as a result of an involuntary dismount, fall of horse and rider, contact with an immobile object such as a gate post, being thrown, or being kicked, bitten or trodden upon when grounded.

Head injuries

No head injury should ever be ignored, however trivial it may seem at the time. The brain is suspended in a water bed inside the skull. The material of the brain, as already described, is highly specialised and very sensitive to compression or bruising. All head injuries must be examined by a doctor and, however inconvenient with regard to curtailment of activity, the advice given must be adhered to. To ignore the advice is just plain stupid; your brain is the central computer, it controls balance, co-ordination, sight, speech and conscious thought as well as every bodily function, reflex or otherwise. You only have one brain: look after it.

Tiresome though it may be to find a skull cap that fits, go on looking. The cap should stay in place when the wearer bends forward, head down, and shakes the head. See that the chin strap fits and is comfortable. Caps with fixed peaks should be avoided. Should a fall occur in such a manner that the peak hits the ground first, the neck will be snapped backwards in an extension movement and a severe whiplash injury will result. Fixed peaks on motorbike helmets were banned years ago because of the problems that they caused.

The effects of a head injury do not always manifest at the time of the accident. Severe headache, any form of blurred vision or other unnatural signs occurring within five days of a fall should be reported to your doctor immediately. There is no possible therapy for a head injury other than rest.

The tempero-mandibular joint

The tempero-mandibular joints are the joints just in front of the ears where the lower jaw is attached to the skull. Falls sometimes sprain and marginally dislodge one or other of the joints. The common symptom is headache, unexplained without reason. Test for a problem in the tempero-mandibular joints by putting your fingers just forward of the middle of the ear, opening the jaw several times and closing it until you can feel the jaw bone move under your fingers. Then apply deep pressure, first on one side of the face and then on the other, over the joint.

If either side is painful, the best advice is to go to see your dentist. Dentists have far more success with problems in this joint than any other therapists.

The shoulder

The shoulder unit consists of the shoulder blade (scapular), the collar bone (clavical) and the upper bone of the arm (humerus).

The shoulder blade and the collar bone join each other at the acromioclavicular joint, a small joint lying just above the shallow saucer on the shoulder blade, which forms the surface for arm movement. Apart from a tiny joint between the breast bone (sternum) and the collar bone, the whole shoulder unit is attached to the body by muscles.

The collar bone

Fractures of the collar bone are common. A figure-of-eight bandage applied to pull both shoulders back will help, and should be used when riding for at least 6–8 weeks after the injury.

The acromioclavicular joint

This joint is usually stressed when the point of the shoulder hits the ground first in a fall. The involvement of the joint is often missed on examination, as the only movement that really stresses the structure is when the arm is taken across the front of the chest, and over-pressure is applied.

The shoulder joint

The joint dislocates when severe traction with rotation occurs – the capsule of the joint, the ligaments and the muscles are all stretched and torn. Occasionally, the large plexus of nerves lying in the armpit, just below the joint, may also be involved. Immobilisation is essential in the early stages after the injury, the most comfortable form being strapping the upper arm to the body.

A frozen shoulder is the term used when the capsule of the joint becomes grossly inflamed; and the arm gets stuck and full movement of the joint is lost. It is a very painful condition and it takes approximately two years to recover untreated. Pain and loss of movement are the predominant features. The condition always does recover, even untreated, but with skilled treatment the pain can be reduced at an early stage.

The elbow

A hinge joint allowing bending and stretching movements, the most usual problems in the elbow are a simple sprain of the joint and tennis or golfer's elbow. Tennis elbow is a tear in the tendon of the muscles that extend the wrist; golfer's elbow is a tear in the tendon of the muscles that flex the wrist.

If the elbow joint is sprained and will not straighten after an accident, avoid straightening. This nearly always results in excess bone formation, and the joint becomes 'fixed'. Should this happen, full movement is lost for good.

The important thing in *any* elbow injury is to achieve full flexion (bending), and this is worth working at. Normally, full extension or straightening will occur over a period of time. It is the forcing of this movement that causes trouble.

Wrist and hand

Sprains of the wrist and finger joints are common. Movement always returns. Occasionally, small bony lumps grow at the site of injury in the joints of the fingers; the periosteum has torn at the time of accident and new bone growth results. These lumps rarely, if ever, affect function.

The hip

Fractures of the head of the femur, the upper bone of the leg, the socket of the joint (the acetabulum) and the shaft of the femur itself are all serious problems requiring medical aid. The most common rider injury is a tear of the adductor muscle causing severe pain in the groin (see Plate 43). Much of other hip and buttock pain experienced is referred from the back.

The knee

The knee is a very complicated joint consisting of two bones, the femur above and the tibia below, with the third bone, the patella, a sesamoid bone contained in the tendon of the large group of muscles that straighten or extend the knee, the quadriceps.

The knee has an intricate ligament and muscle arrangement. Most usually torn are the ligaments lying on the inner aspect of the knee or the ligament running round the joint. Tears of the latter may involve a cartilage. Knee cartilages do not heal and bad tears usually require surgical intervention. Modern techniques allow the insertion of a small camera into the joint to assess the interior damage. Small pieces of cartilage that are torn can be removed by this technique, known as 'arthroscopy'.

Rotational stress of the knee often causes severe bleeds into the joint, with associated swelling and pain.

The ankle

The outer side of the ankle takes the strain on rough ground when the ankle 'turns over'. Swelling, pain and loss of movement are the immediate results.

The foot

Severe bruising and even bone damage occur when the full weight of a horse's foot falls on any part of the human. The foot is particularly vulnerable but fortunately, given time, mends well.

Types of injury

Fracture equals broken bone. Fractures are caused by direct trauma such as being kicked, as a result of a fall when the bone is stressed unacceptably, or as the result of a rotational strain.

Bone mends well, provided the broken pieces are held correctly aligned. Manipulative reduction under anaesthetic is usually required in cases of major breaks, followed by immobilisation in a plaster or fibreglass cast.

Simple breaks in fingers do well strapped with adhesive tape; severe, unstable breaks may require pinning or plating. Recovery takes 4–6 weeks in the case of a simple break, but more severe problems can take several months. Immobilisation of the collar bone, shoulder blade or ribs is very difficult and these bones are usually left to heal as best they can. The ribs can cause problems if they fracture and the pieces bend inward, piercing a part of the lung. If rib fracture is suspected, X-rays should always be taken.

Dislocation

Dislocation occurs when the bones comprising a joint are pulled apart and fail to return to their normal anatomical position. The capsule is stretched and torn, as are the ligaments and the muscles of the joint. Immediately dislocation occurs, the supporting muscles go into strong spasm and it is usually impossible to re-align the bones of the joint without anaesthesia.

Strains and sprains

The terminology for overstretch of ligamentous tissue is 'strain'. Overstretched ligaments, when associated with a joint, reduce the stability of the joint.

The terminology for an overstretched joint that is not dislocated is 'sprain'. Joints are sprained when they are put through a movement range greater than they are designed to perform.

Muscle

Muscle fibres, being highly elastic, are fairly resilient to stress. Problems occur at the point where the muscle is attached to bone: sudden exertion rips the attachment. Muscles in 'peak condition' sometimes rupture spontaneously, tears in the muscle belly occurring due to a sudden unexpected change of function. For example, a person is leading a horse, elbow bent; the horse suddenly rears and pulls back, the elbow is straightened sharply; the sudden and unexpected force tears the biceps muscle, the main elbow flexor, because at the time of the unexpected movement the muscle fibres were in a state of contraction – they were not relaxed.

Bruises

Bruises are caused by the seepage of blood from tiny vessels injured at the time of an accident. The blood cells free in the tissue cause chemical reactions and discoloration, the colour of the bruise changing as the body responds to the unusual situation and begins to break down and re-absorb the effects of the damage. The greater the blood seepage, the larger and more painful the bruise.

Self help

It is nearly impossible to be involved in any sport without the odd injury occurring, and association with the horse is no exception. Sportsmen in all other disciplines seek qualified professional help from their doctor, physiotherapist or trainer after injury, and return to their sport fully fit and *pain free*. Not so members of the equestrian fraternity, who must constitute the largest group of DIY healers within the world of sport.

This short section is not an attempt to teach 'DIY healing', but rather to suggest which methods to choose if you, the injured, prefer to 'chance it' rather than be treated professionally. Guidelines are difficult. Each case differs in so many ways – in the main, if the machine causes pain you have either chosen the wrong machine or the setting is incorrect. The line of thought 'it's hurting me, it must be doing good' is nonsense – and is a dangerous attitude, particularly when using ultrasound. Pain means you are burning, damaging or destroying tissue, the very reverse of what is required. So what can be used safely from the horse repair kit?

Fractures

Recent work indicates that repair of bone is enhanced by the use of magnetic fields. It is safe to use the machines *unless* the break has necessitated the use of pins or plates. Treatment should *not* cause pain.

There is always deterioration of muscle after a fracture, and it is of the utmost importance to maintain muscle strength. Unfortunately, muscles loose their 'tone' very rapidly and are slow to rebuild. Move the joints above and below the cast as much as is possible. If fingers or toes are exposed, move them. Try to tighten and relax the muscles inside the cast – this helps to maintain muscle but also, even more important, aids circulatory flow. Remember, no healing can take place without an adequate circulation. When the cast is removed, if you have a muscle stimulator, use it.

The weaker muscles will *never* catch up with their stronger brothers unless exercised separately. Groups of muscles, weaker than they should be, create the situation of imbalance with consequent uneven stress on the joints involved, leading to problems years after the injury occurred.

Dislocation

Pain, swelling and loss of movement are all present. Cold and massage will help the swelling and ease the pain. If the joint is immobilised, tighten and relax all the muscles around the joint. Just as with a fracture, this will retain muscle strength, aid circulatory flow and aid healing.

The maintenance of muscle strength after dislocation is of the utmost importance, for the stretched ligaments will never completely recover their original size and strength; therefore the joint will depend on muscle strength for stability. The magnetic field machine, ultrasound, massage and muscle stimulation will all be of use post dislocation.

Sprains and strains

The usual pattern of pain, swelling and loss of movement is present. Reduce the swelling with cold and massage. Cold bandages, especially the Bonner types with their inbuilt elastic support, are very useful.

Magnetic field and ultrasound will help the swelling to reduce, but used too early the machines will not be of use – always wait for 24–48 hours. Should the swelling or pain increase after treatment, you have started too early and/or are using the wrong settings.

Muscle tears

The earlier gentle movement is started, the less scarring in the tissues and the better the end result. Reduce the swelling and help the pain with cold. Use the ultrasound on a very low setting and use the muscle stimulator.

Bruises

Cold, massage and magnetic field therapy are the most useful in the early stages. Large haematomas will benefit from ultrasound after 2–3 days.

General rehabilitation

Contrary to the ideas of many people, riding a horse does not make you fit. Mr Thelwell produced a brilliant drawing titled 'The Body Beautiful – What Three Months' Riding Can Do', the drawing depicting a very fat lady bumping along on a very fat horse. On the next page, titled 'After', the picture showed the very fat lady now on a very thin horse! Fit horse, still-fat lady.

All winning riders are immensely conscious of the need to be fit, working out in gyms and swimming pools, jogging, and riding bikes (the latter best without the saddle). Getting fit is, to many, a bore; regaining fitness after injury is even worse – but remember that injury, although confined in many cases to a small area, affects the working of the entire body. Injuries recover quicker given, first, treatment and specific work for tissues in the area involved, followed by a programme of general activity.

The principles of the repair programme are the same for rider and horse: aid the repair after damage, regain full movement and muscle strength and re-educate the whole to regain confidence.

Appendix I
Bandaging

Whatever the reason for bandaging, be it for support while working, support after injury, pressure for reduction of swelling or warmth, the basic problem is to apply the bandage in such a way that it is functionally useful, does not slip and does not interfere with circulatory flow.

There are many types of materials on the market, and only common sense can dictate the tension required for each type to enable the bandage to fulfil an adequate function. The emphasis when bandaging must be on evenness of tension; however soft the body of the material, an overtight edge or overtight turn can cause major damage to the underlying tissues. The tendons and joints of the legs are particularly vulnerable to damage from lumps, creases, overtight bandages, or bandages left in situ for too long.

Gamgee or some other suitable padding material wrapped carefully around the leg under the bandage gives a better distribution of pressure, but care must be taken not to overrun the edge of the padding. The longer the bandage, the more gradual the spiral and the less likelihood of damage from creases.

A well rolled bandage is a must. It is far easier to get even pressure by carefully unrolling the bandage round the leg. If the bandage ties with tapes, the tapes should be kept flat and must not be pulled tight; they must be at the same tension as the bandage. If crepe or tapeless bandages that do not have velcro fastenings are used, the best way to secure is with a strip of adhesive tape, micropore or elastoplast.

Extra care must be taken when bandaging the knee joint. The accessory carpal bone (piseform) protrudes at the back of the knee, and is especially susceptible to pressure. A figure-of-eight type bandage should therefore be used, this giving minimal pressure over the accessory carpal bone.

Types of bandage

Tube gauze: an elasticated stocking sleeve useful for supporting underlying dressings. Available in various widths from all the larger pharmacies.

Glentona bandages: made of a thermolactic material whose properties include the ability for moisture to pass from the inner to the outer surface of the bandage.

Coldwrap: these are an impregnated gauze, the chemical remaining cold for up to six hours when exposed to air. They can be re-rolled and kept in an airtight plastic container in the refrigerator and re-used.

Crepe bandages: most satisfactory for support and pressure. If rinsed in warm water after use, will regain their elasticity. Without their elasticity, they are of no benefit and can be dangerous.

Wet bandages: some bandages shrink as they dry; this can cause a severe reduction in blood flow, damage to the skin and underlying structures. Use with great care.

Bandages, whatever their function (unless ordered to be left in place by the veterinary surgeon), should be removed at least every 12 hours. When removed, a quick hand massage will stimulate the skin circulation. Allow the area to breathe. When the bandages are re-applied, care should be taken to ensure the folds lie in such a way that the edges of the bandage cover a different area.

Appendix II
Cupping

Adherent scar is often very difficult to free from the underlying tissues, particularly after injuries to the front of the knee, the scar tending to split on the resumption of activity requiring full knee flexion.

Cupping was the old fashioned method of raising the skin from the underlying tissues. Used with blood letting or the application of leeches (!), the apparatus consisted of a small short glass or bone funnel with a rubber ball fixed over the narrow end. The open end was placed firmly on a patch of dampened skin. By squeezing the rubber ball, air was evacuated; the ball was released slowly and the vacuum created pulled the underlying skin into the funnel aperture, thus stretching the tissue.

Exactly the same effect can be obtained by cutting the end off a 5 cc syringe; the open end is placed on the scar, which must be damp or oiled, and the plunger is then withdrawn. The tissue lying beneath the syringe is drawn up the barrel. Underlying adhesions can be stretched and the scar, if adherent, freed.

It must be remembered that scar tissue has virtually no blood supply, and care must be taken to ensure that there is no damage to the few blood vessels that are present.

Appendix III
Points for Those Treating Horses

Retain a professional approach and appearance. The animal may not be fussy – but animals have owners!

Wear clothes that do not restrict movement. You may have to kneel for long periods or move suddenly at speed.

Wear a kennel coat: the pockets are invaluable. Unless you have a purpose built unit in a veterinary yard, you will be working in a grooming or loose box. It is sometimes possible to use a straw-bale table; if not, there is just the floor. Vital leads have a habit of getting lost in bedding, so use pockets.

Boots are more useful than shoes. Make certain they have good, non-slip soles. Some are designed with steel toe caps – very useful, as toes break easily if stamped on. Boots do not fill with bedding, and you do not make a neatly swept yard messy by trailing bedding or shavings as you leave the box.

Avoid wearing jewellery. Rings have a habit of catching, and many people have broken fingers by getting rings caught.

Use a good-sized watch that can be read easily and is waterproof.

Perfume upsets some animals – their smell appreciation differs from ours. (A notice on a monkey cage stated: 'We can smell you too, you know!')

Machines

If possible, have a strong outer box made for each machine. Ultrasound machines do not like being kicked or trodden on. A compartment within the box for leads, gels, etc., is a great advantage.

General points

Make certain all machines are turned back to zero before switching on. A patient will tell you if something has happened; a horse will kick you if all is not well. Test on yourself before using – once you have frightened an animal, it takes a long time for him to regain confidence.

Stables are sparsely provided with plugs, so take at least two long extension leads with you, 5 metres in length. Battery operated machines are preferable.

Keep all lotions, solvents and gels in plastic containers: broken glass is a disaster. A bucket is a useful carrier for pads, electrodes, spare leads, sponges, salt, towels and other necessities. You will need a second bucket for soaking pads.

Have an adjustable rope halter with you in case you arrive and find the tack room locked or all halters in use.

A plastic bib can be useful: if you have a patient that bites at one end and kicks at the other, you can eliminate one danger! Machines with leads attached to specialised pads are a hazard; it is amazing how quickly leads can be chewed through, and bandages or boots removed. The bib prevents this.

Carry a tape measure and a pair of carpenter's dividers. These allow you to record accurate measurement of swelling in the limb or the muscle bulk of the forelimb or hindlimb. The length from the bulb of the heel to the heel of the shoe is also worth measuring. There is very often great disparity between the inner and the outer side of the heel, and this can be a cause of breakdown. Owners accept measurement, not guess work.

Carry a clip board with attached pad for recording case histories. Your case histories must be accurate. Polaroid or other photographs are a useful record.

A plastic milk crate makes a useful platform if a horse is taller than you. It can also be used as a table or stool. Most dairies will sell you one. (N.B. Some makes are stronger than others.)

The owner

Owners are often very emotionally involved with their animals. The mere fact that the animal is ill or injured, and that they might themselves have contributed to the injury, may make them feel helpless, frustrated and even angry. This may result in their being quite unable to help and irrational about suggestions made.

Explain what is going to be done and why, and also the possible reaction of the animal, including the effects of and reaction to the treatments: some treatments make the situation worse before it gets better.

Discuss aftercare; write down what the owner or groom is to do between visits. If called to a big yard, find out the yard routine – in hospitals, all treatments fit in with ward routine, and so should your visits.

In a racing yard, the head lad is very important. Make yourself known to him; without his help and backing, you may just as well go home, whatever the owner or trainer says. The head lad will respect you for your knowledge if you respect him for his, and will ensure that any requests for specialist exercise or grooming are carried out.

The lad who does and rides the horse will be a mine of useful information, so talk to him.

Appendix IV
The Use of Anti-Concussion Pads

Shock and vibration and the associated musculoskeletal problems which they promote in the human have long been studied, and are accepted and well documented. The ability to measure by means of 'force plates' the impact shock or 'G' created when the foot meets the ground has led to the development of new types of material designed to dissipate the 'G' force by as much as 78 per cent.

The musculoskeletal structure of the horse is subjected to forces ranging from 30 G at the walk to as much as 360 G galloping and jumping – that is, the limb first touching the ground after the suspension phase at gallop, or landing after a jump, sustains a load equivalent to 360 times the normal body weight of the animal. Small wonder that such force creates problems in the foot and lower leg.

While it may be argued that the majority of the impact is absorbed by the digital cushion and some by the natural expansion and flexibility of the hoof, not all is accounted for and shock waves proceed up the leg until they finally terminate in the spine. The amount of shock dissipated in the foot is also dependent on the foot being correctly trimmed, the balance between the toe and heel, the fit of the shoe – in short, good foot care.

Polyurethane and visco elastic polymer are first cousins, designed with a molecular structure that is able to absorb and dissipate shock laterally (sideways), thus reducing the G force sustained by the landing foot by as much as 78 per cent. Riders using these pads (Plate 44) have reported that their horses felt more comfortable and moved more freely. While this is a subjective observation, the level of rider questioned would indicate honest appraisal.

The pads are available in different degrees of thickness, the choice dependent upon the disciplines of the horse. Available as rims or full pads, they are fitted under the shoe. As the material is able to breathe, no problems associated with the sole being covered have yet been encountered.

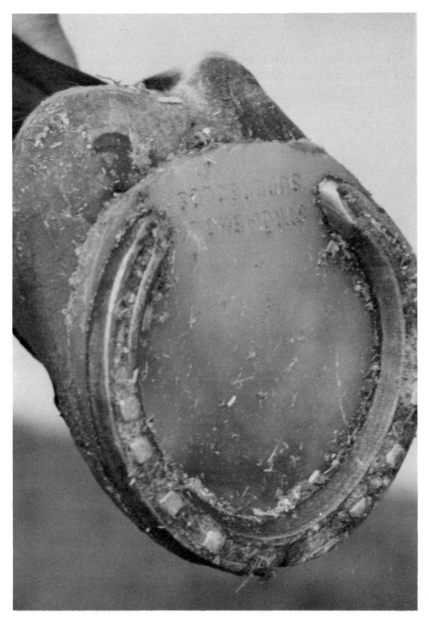

Plate 44 Anti-concussion pad designed to dissipate the shock to the landing foot by as much as 78 per cent.

Glossary

Abdomen: that portion of the body which lies between the chest and the pelvis.

Abduction: a drawing away from the median plane of the body.

Absorption: the uptake of substances into or across tissues.

Acute: having a short and relatively severe course.

Adduction: a drawing towards the median plane of the body.

Adhesion: a fibrous band abnormally joining tissues together.

Adrenaline: an important hormone secreted by the medulla of the adrenal gland.

Aerobic: growing in the presence of oxygen.

Analgesic: relieving pain.

Anaemia: a below normal number of erythrocytes per mm^2, or in the quantity of haemoglobin, which occurs when the equilibrium between blood loss and blood production is disturbed.

Anterior: situated in front of, or in the forward part of, an organ; towards the head end of the body.

Antiseptic: an agent that prevents the decay or decomposition of tissue by inhibiting the growth and development of micro-organisms.

Anus: the external opening of the rectum.

Aorta: the main artery of the arterial system which carries blood away from the heart.

Arteriole: a minute arterial branch, especially one near a capillary.

Artery: vessel through which blood passes away from the heart towards the various parts of the body.

Arthritis: inflammation of joints.

Articular: pertaining to, divided by, or united by joints.

Ataxia: an inability to co-ordinate voluntary muscular movements.

Atrophy: wasting away of a normally developed organ or tissue due to degeneration of cells.

Avascular: not supplied with blood vessels.

Avulsion: the tearing away of part of a structure.

Bifurcation: the site where a single structure divides into two branches.

Bilateral: having two sides or pertaining to both sides.

Blistering: applying an agent to the skin to produce blistering and inflammation of the skin; used to treat chronic or subacute inflammation of joints, tendons, and bones.

Blood pressure: the pressure of blood on the walls of the arteries, dependent on the energy of the heart action, the elasticity of the walls of the arteries, and the volume and viscosity of the blood.

Bog spavin: a chronic distension of the joint capsule of the hock with synovial fluid.

Bone spavin: a lameness, originating in the hock, which is characterised by either exostosis or bone destruction on the inner surface of the hock.

Bowed tendon: damage to the tendon that results in inflammation.

Broken wind: an inability to empty the lungs of air, caused by the rupture of some alveoli, and characterised by difficult breathing, a chronic cough, and generally poor condition.

Bronchial: pertaining to either or both of the two main branches of the trachea, one going to each lung.

Bronchus, bronchi: either or both of the two main branches of the trachea, one going to each lung.

Bucked shins: a periostitis of the front side of the cannon bone; usually occuring on the forelegs of young horses that are strenuously exercised.

Bursa: a sac or sac-like cavity filled with fluid and situated at places in the tissues at which friction would otherwise develop.

Bursitis: an inflammation of the bursa, occasionally accompanied by the formation of a calcific deposit in the underlying tendon.

Calcification: the process of tissue becoming hardened by a deposit of calcium salts.

Callus: localised hyperplasia of the epidermis due to friction or pressure; an unorganised woven meshwork of bone which forms at the site of a fracture and is eventually replaced by hard adult bone.

Capped elbow: a soft, flabby swelling over the point of the elbow due to trauma.

Capped hock: an inflammation of the bursa over the point of the hock caused by trauma.

Cardiac: pertaining to the heart.

Cardiac cycle: the actions of the heart during one complete heart beat.

Carpal: pertaining to the knee.

Chronic: long term, continued, not acute.

Clot: a semi-solidified mass of blood.

Collagen: a main fibrous protein of skin, bone, tendon, cartilage and connective tissue.

Collateral: secondary or accessory; a small side branch, as of a blood vessel or nerve.

Concussion: a violent jar or shock.

Conformation: the shape or contour of the body or body structures.

Congenital: existing at and usually before birth; referring to conditions that may or may not be inherited.

Connective tissue: the tissue which binds together and is the support of the various structures of the body.

Contusion: a bruise or injury incurred without breaking the skin.

Cow hocks: a conformation fault in which the hocks are pointed inward when viewed from behind.

Curb: a thickening of the plantar tarsal ligament, resulting in an enlargement below the point of the hock, and marked by inflammation and lameness.

Dehydration: condition resulting from excessive loss of body water.

Diagnosis: distinguishing one disease from another, or identifying a disease from its characteristics and/or causative agent.

Diaphragm: the muscular membrane separating the abdominal and chest cavities.

Digital: pertaining to the long and short pastern bones and the coffin bone.

Dilatation: the condition of being dilated or stretched beyond normal dimensions.

Dilation: a stretching or expansion.

Dislocation: the displacement of any part, usually referring to a bone.

Distal: a point further from the centre of the body.

Distension: the state of being swollen or enlarged from internal pressure.

Dorsal: pertaining to the back or denoting a position more towards the back surface than some other point of reference.

Dysfunction: disturbance or impairing of the function of an organ.

Electrolyte: a substance present in body fluids which is capable of conducting electricity in various body functions such as nerve impulses, oxygen and carbon dioxide transport, and muscle contraction.

Epidermis: the outermost layer of skin which is not supplied with blood vessels.

Epiphysis: a part of a bone, especially at the end of a long bone, which develops separately from the shaft of the bone during the growth period – during this time it is separated from the main portion of the bone by cartilage.

Epiphysitis: inflammation of the end of a long bone or of the cartilage that separates it from the long bone.

Epithelium: the covering of internal and external surfaces of the body, including the lining of vessels and other small cavities; it consists of cells joined together by small amounts of cementing substances.

Extension: a movement that brings a limb into a straight line.

Extensor: any muscle that extends a joint.

Facet: a small plane or surface on a hard body, as on a bone.

Fascia: a sheet or band of fibrous tissue lying below the skin or surrounding muscles and various organs of the body.

Fetlock: the area or joint of the lower leg above the pastern and below the cannon.

Fibrosis: the formation of fibrous tissue.

Fibrous adhesion: a fibrous band or structure by which parts abnormally adhere.

Filing: the act of filing down the teeth to remove sharp edges; also referred to as floating.

Flexion: the act of bending.

Fossa: a hollow or depressed area.

Fracture: the breaking of a part, especially a bone.

Frog: the band of horny substance in the middle of the sole of a horse's foot, dividing into two branches and running towards the heel in the shape of a 'V'.

Gaskin: the thigh of a horse.

Gastric: pertaining to the stomach.

Haematoma: an accumulation of blood within the tissues that clots to form a solid swelling.

Haemoglobin: the oxygen-carrying protein pigment of the red blood cells.

Haemorrhage: the escape of blood from the vessels; bleeding.

Hoof tester: a pincer-like instrument used to gently squeeze the hoofs to find any sore areas; if this is done in an area of inflammation the horse will flinch.

Hyperextend: extreme or excessive extension of a limb.

Hyperflexion: forcible overflexion of a limb or part.

Hypersensitivity: a state of altered activity in which the body reacts with an exaggerated response to a foreign agent.

Insertion: the point of attachment of a muscle (e.g. to a bone).

Inspiration: the act of inhaling or drawing air into the lungs.

Intravenous: within a vein.

Involuntary: performed independently of the will, contravolitional; as in an involuntary muscle.

Ischaemia: inadequate circulatory flow caused by constriction of the local blood vessels.

Joint: an articulation; the place of union or junction between two or more bones of the skeleton.

Laceration: a torn, ragged wound.

Laminitis: inflammation of a lamina, especially the laminae of a horse's foot.

Larynx: the structure of muscle and cartilage located at the top of the trachea and below the root of the tongue; 'voice box'.

Lateral: pertaining to a side or outer surface; a position further from the midline of the body or of a structure.

Lesion: an abnormal change in the structure of a part due to injury or disease.

Ligament: a band of fibrous tissue that connects bones or cartilages.

Lumbar: pertaining to the loins, the part of the back between the thorax and pelvis.

Luxation: dislocation.

Lymph: a transparent yellowish liquid containing mostly white blood cells and derived from tissue fluids.

Medial: pertaining to the middle or inner surface; a position closer to the midline of the body or of a structure.

Metatarsal: cannon; the area between the hock and fetlock joint.

Mobility: the ability to move.

Muscle: an organ which by contraction produces the movements of an animal organism.

Muscle tremor: an involuntary trembling or quivering of a muscle.

Navicular: a small bone in the foot of a horse; common term to designate pathology of the navicular bone.

Necrosis: death of a cell or group of cells which is in contact with living tissue.

Nerves: cord-like structures, visible to the naked eye, comprising a collection of nerve fibres which convey impulses between a part of the central nervous system and some other region of the body.

Non-vascular: not supplied with blood vessels.

Oedema: excessive accumulation of fluid in the body tissues.

Olecranon: the point of the elbow formed by the bony projection of the ulna.

Optic: pertaining to the eye.

Origin: the point of attachment of a muscle that remains relatively fixed during contraction of the muscle.

Ossify: to change or develop into bone.

Palpation: the act of feeling with the hand.

Pastern: the area between the fetlock joint and the coronary band.

Patella: a triangular sesamoid bone situated at the front of the stifle; also called the knee cap.

Pathological: a diseased condition.

Pelvis: the rear portion of the trunk of the body, bounded by the hip bones.

Peripheral circulatory system: the part of the circulatory system that carries blood to the outer parts of the body such as the legs.

Phalanx: any of the three bones below the fetlock: the long pastern bone, short pastern bone, and coffin bone.

Plasma: the liquid portion of the blood, containing the suspended particulate components.

Platelets: disc-shaped structures found in the blood of all mammals and chiefly known for their role in the blood coagulation; also called blood platelets. (See also *Thrombocytes.*)

Plexus: a network of lymphatic vessels, nerves, veins, or arteries.

Posterior: situated behind, or in the back of, a structure; towards the rear end of the body.

Poultice: a soft, moist, mass of the consistency of cooked cereal, spread between layers of muslin, linen, gauze, or towels, and applied hot to a given area in order to create moist local heat or counter-irritation.

Prognosis: the prospect of recovery from a disease or injury.

Progressive: advancing, going from bad to worse; advancing in severity.

Proud flesh: excessive granulation tissue.

Proximal: a point near to the centre of the body.

Pulmonary: pertaining to the lungs.

Pulse: rhythmic throbbing of an artery which may be felt with the finger; caused by blood forced through the vessel by contractions of the heart.

Pus: a liquid inflammation product made up of leucocytes and a thin fluid called liquor puris.

Rasping: filing the teeth with a rasp to provide dental care.

Red blood cells: haemoglobin-carrying corpuscles in the blood that transport oxygen.

Reflex arc: the neural arc used in a reflex action.

Regeneration: the natural renewal of a structure, as of a tissue part.

Ringbone: a general term that applies to bony enlargements and areas of new bone growth below the fetlock.

Roach back: a conformation fault in which the back is arched and convex. This fault predisposes a horse to forging and shortens the gait of the animal.

Rotation: the process of turning around an axis.

Rupture: a breaking or tearing of tissue.

Sacrioliac: pertaining to the sacrum and ilium, denoting the joint or articulation between the sacrum and ilium and associated ligaments.

Sacrum: the triangular bone just below the lumbar vetebrae, wedged dorsally between the two wings of the hip bone.

Saddle sore: a simple inflammation of hair follicles (usually on the withers) caused by friction between the horse and the saddle.

Sand cracks: cracks in the hoof wall.

Scar tissue: tissue remaining after the healing of a wound or other morbid process.

Sebaceous: a thick, fatty semifluid substance secreted by the skin.

Seedy toe: a disease of the hoof wall in the toe region in which the hoof wall is separated from the white line.

Septum: a dividing wall or partition.

Sequestra: pieces of dead bone that have been broken off or become separated, during the process of necrosis, from the sound bone.

Sesamoid: a small nodular bone embedded in a tendon or joint capsule.

Sesamoiditis: an inflammation of the proximal sesamoid bones, usually involving both osteitis and periostitis.

Shin buck: See *Bucked shins.*

Sickle hocks: deviations in the angle of the hock as seen from the side; the cannon slopes forward due to excessive angulation of the hock.

Sinusitis: inflammation of a sinus, marked by discharge of pus from one or both nostrils.

Spasm: a sudden, involuntary contraction of a muscle or constriction of a passage.

Spavin test: a test in which the affected leg is held acutely flexed for about two minutes, then released immediately before the horse is trotted; the test is considered positive for bone spavin if lameness is markedly increased for the horse's first few steps.

Splints: rigid or flexible appliances for the fixation of displaced or movable parts.

Sprain: a joint injury in which some of the fibres of a ligament are ruptured.

Strain: an overstretching or overexertion of some part of the musculature.

Stress: forcibly exerted influence or pressure.

Subacute: somewhat acute, between acute and chronic.

Subluxation: an incomplete or partial dislocation.

Supraspinous: above a spine or spinous process.

Suspensory: a ligament, bone, muscle, sling or bandage which holds up a part.

Synovial fluid: a transparent fluid, resembling the white of an egg, secreted by the synovial membrane and contained in joint cavities, bursae and tendon sheaths for lubrication.

Tendon: a fibrous cord of connective tissue which attaches muscle to bone or other structures.

Thorax, thoracic: the chest; the part of the body between the neck and the diaphragm, encased by the ribs.

Thrombocytes: blood platelets.

Tied in at the knee: a condition occurring when the flexor tendons appear to be too close to the cannon bone just below the knee.

Tissue: an aggregation of similarly specialised cells united in the performance of a particular function.

Trauma: a wound or injury.

Ultrasonics: the use of controlled doses of high frequency sound (radiation) for therapeutic treatment.

Vein: a vessel through which the blood passes from various organs or parts back to the heart.

Venous: pertaining to the veins.

Voluntary: accomplished in accordance with the will.

Windgalls: also called windpuffs; a distention (overfilling) of the synovial sheath between the suspensory ligament and the cannon bone, or of the synovial sheath between the long pastern and the middle inferior sesamoidean ligament.

Wobbler: a disease that affects the cervical spinal cord and vetebrae of young horses; it is a sporadic, non-paralytic condition marked by inco-ordination. Also known as equine inco-ordination.

Bibliography

Anatomy

Adams, O. R. (1974) *Lameness in Horses*. 3rd Ed. USA: Lea and Febiger.

De Lahunta, Alexander, DVM, PhD (1983) *Veterinary Neuroanatomy and Clinical Neurology*. 2nd Ed. W. B. Saunders Co.

Goody, Peter C., BSc, PhD (1976) *Horse Anatomy*. J. A. Allen.

Green, Ben K. (1982) *Horse Conformation as to Soundness and Performance*. Northland Press.

Le Vay, David (1974) *Human Anatomy and Physiology*. Hodder and Stoughton

Luard, Lowes D. (1935) *The Horse Its Action and Anatomy by an Artist*. Faber & Faber Ltd.

Lumley, J. S. P., Craven, J. L., Aitken, J. T. (1975) *Essential Anatomy*. Churchill Livingstone.

Sisson and Grossman (1975) *The Anatomy of the Domestic Animals*. Vols 1 and 2. 3rd Ed. W. B. Saunders Co.

Stubbs, George (1976) *The Anatomy of the Horse*. New York: Dover Publications, Inc.

Treatment

Downer, Ann H., BA, MA, LPT (1978) *Physical Therapy for Animals Selected Techniques*. Illinois: Charles C. Thomas.

Forster, A. and Palastanga, N. (1981) *Clayton's Electrotherapy*. Balliere Tindall.

Lee, Jennifer, M. and Warren, Margaret, P. (1978) *Cold Therapy in Rehabilitation*. Bell and Hyman.

Meagher, Jack (1986) *Beating Muscle Injuries for Horses*. Ref. *Equus magazine*. J. A. Allen.

Westermayer, Erwin, Dr Med Vet (1979) *The Treatment of Horses by Acupuncture*. Health Science Press.

Schooling for rehabilitation

Becher, Rolf (1963) *Schooling by the Natural Method*. J. A. Allen.
de Ruffieu, Francois Lemaire (1986) *The Handbook of Riding Essentials*. New York: Harper & Row Publishers.
Ivers, Tom (1983) *The Fit Racehorse*. Ohio: Espirit Racing Team Ltd.
Oliveira, Nuno (1983) *Classical Principles of the Art of Training Horses*. Australia: Howley and Russell.
Richards, P. K. (1983) *The BLOK Training System*. Richard's Bloks Ltd.
Swift, Sally (1985) *Centered Riding*. Vermont: A Trafalgar Farm Book, David and Charles Inc.
Wilson, Gary, L. DVM, Mueller, Martha (1982) *The Equine Athlete*. USA: Veterinary Learning Systems.

Kinesiology

Rooney, James R., DVM (1980) *The Mechanics of the Horse*. New York: Robert E. Krieger Publishing Co. Inc.
Smith, R. N. (1983) *The Locomotor System*. Dept. of Anatomy, University of Bristol.
Smythe, R. H., MRCVS (1975) *The Horse Structure and Movement*. 2nd Edn. J. A. Allen.
Wynmalen, Henry (1954) *The Horse in Action*. Harold Starke Ltd.

Farriery

Hogg, Garry (1964) *Hammer and Tongs*. Hutchinson.
(1975) *The Horses's Foot: A guide for A.F.C.L. Students*. CoSIRA.

Reference/Encyclopaedia

Cailliet, Rene, MD (1977) *Soft Tissue Pain & Disability*. Philadelphia: F. A. Davis Co.
Equine Research (1977) *Veterinary Encyclopaedia for Horsemen*. Don. M. Wagoner.
Lyon, W. E., Lt Col (1966) *First Aid Hints for the Horse Owner*. 10th Edn. London: Collins.
Miller, W. C. and West, G. P. (1959) *Black's Veterinary Dictionary*. A. & C. Black.
Sperryn, Peter N. (1983) *Sport and Medicine*. Butterworths.
Summerhays, R. S. (1966) *Summerhays' Encyclopaedia for Horsemen*. Frederick Warne & Co. Ltd.

Index